Praise for *The Whole Body S*

'Although we have had great exploratic
the wonders of the human body. Nine 1
supporting cast allow you to breathe, th
human in this universe of endless possib........

'Max Tuck brings you into this world in a way that has never been done before. I strongly advise you to strap in and enjoy the ride.'

Dr Brian Clement PhD, LN
Director, Hippocrates Health Institute, Florida

'Beautifully clear and concise, Max has tackled this enormous subject scientifically but without jargon. As I read each sentence, I could hear Max presenting it all as one of her excellent, humorous, illustrated lectures. As an extremely busy small-animal veterinary surgeon, an athlete and a most knowledgeable nutritionist, Max absolutely walks her talk. Everything she says in her books and presentations, she does! She is the busiest, most energetic person I know, with a fantastic figure, amazing skin and the most beautiful hair I have ever seen and she is 100% fuelled by raw vegan food. If you want even a fraction of what she has, read and digest this wonderful book and follow her recommendations to the letter!'

Suzi McIntyre BVSc, MRCVS, DNN
Naturopathic Nutritionist, Founding President of BVDA

'Nothing is more important than gaining insight and wisdom into how you function at your personal best. In this book Max Tuck unveils a practical blueprint that you can use immediately.

'Lifestyle governs everything, and as you upgrade your lifestyle with a healthy mix of fun- and easy-to-digest science, your life will surely never be the same again. Whether you want simple solutions or more complex answers – *The Whole Body Solution* puts you in the driving seat.'

Mike Nash
Director, Aggressive Health Ltd, UK

'Every time I talk to Max, even in a social environment, I learn something new because she has a special knack in bringing science to our everyday experiences in a very practical way. Now she has composed her third book to educate us further in understanding how the various systems work in our body. Of course, I can praise her depth of knowledge, but what particularly stands out from Max's works is the beauty of her written word. Indeed, Max's wit and eloquent explanations make this book an utter joy to read and you get educated as an extra bonus! This marriage between easy, beautiful prose and science results in the perfect choice for both seekers of advanced information and beginners who look for entertainment with interesting facts they can apply to their health path. The only question remains: what will you delight us with next, Max?'

Rian Torres
Director of Health Etcetera

To Talib.
Enjoy the
benefits!
Love,
Max

THE
WHOLE BODY
SOLUTION

Max Tuck
aka The Raw Food Scientist

with a Foreword by
Sarah Best

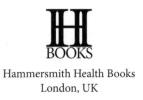

Hammersmith Health Books
London, UK

First published in 2014 by Hammersmith Health Books – an imprint of
Hammersmith Books Limited
14 Greville Street, London EC1N 8SB, UK
www.hammersmithbooks.co.uk

The information contained in this book is for educational purposes only.
It is the result of the study and the experience of the author. Whilst the
information and advice offered are believed to be true and accurate at
the time of going to press. neither the author nor the publisher can accept
any legal responsibility or liability for any errors or omissions that may
have been made or for any adverse effects which may occur as a result of
following the recommendations given herein. Always consult a qualified
medical practitioner if you have any concerns regarding your health.

British Library Cataloguing in Publication Data: A CIP record of this book
is available from the British Library.

Print ISBN 978-1-78161-043-5
Ebook ISBN 978-1-78161-044-2

Commissioning editor: Georgina Bentliff
Designed and typeset by: Julie Bennett
Cover design by: Stewart Lynch
Index: Dr Laurence Errington
Production: Helen Whitehorn, Pathmedia
Printed and bound by: TJ International Ltd

Contents

About me and my contributors

Max Tuck, aka 'The Raw Food Scientist'

I trained in veterinary medicine and come to all health issues, both human and animal, with a rigorously scientific approach. Now a Hippocrates Institute-trained health educator as well as a practising vet, I was originally prompted to investigate the importance of nutrition to health by my own collapse with chronic fatigue and Epstein Barr virus more than 20 years ago. Since my 'miraculous' recovery I have run marathons, competed in triathlons and gained my black belt in karate, in addition to managing my punishing dual-role work schedule. Visit me at www.therawfoodscientist.com.

My contributors

Sarah Best

Sarah Best studied at the College of Natural Nutrition, and has since written and published thousands of articles on all aspects of health and nutrition. She was the editor of *Get Fresh!* magazine from 2006 to 2011, in which capacity she worked with the world's leading experts on holistic health and optimum nutrition. She is now an author and health coach.

www.sarahbesthealth.com

Judy Barber

With a BEd in English, psychology and education, and certificates in Drama Therapy, NLP Practitioner Level, Newcastle College Performance Coaching and Fraser Clarke Business Coaching, Judy has been self-employed as a coach, facilitator and writer since 2003. In 2008 she trained as a Hippocrates Health Educator and has added wellness coaching, particularly around raw and living vegetarian food, to her already impressive CV.

Author of the excellent recipe book *Good Raw Food Recipes*, Judy believes we can 'have it all' by finding balance, bringing our own dreams into reality and giving to life. People choose to work with Judy to achieve personal, career and business goals and when they want their lives to matter. Judy is based in Gloucestershire in the UK.

www.judy-barber.com

Jessica Li

Jessica Li, BA, CRC, CPT (ACSM), is a raw food chef and certified personal trainer based in Toronto, Ontario, Canada. She is known as the 'Supercharged Fitness Coach', and offers raw food classes, women's and corporate personal training, and holistic retreats to clients around the world. She is also the owner of Chica Momma Health and Juice Bar in Toronto.

www.thesuperchargedfitnesscoach.com
www.chicamomma.com

Karen Ranzi

Author, lecturer, health coach, raw vegan chef and speech pathologist, Karen Ranzi, MA, authored and published her book *Creating Healthy Children* in 2010. Her upcoming book, *Raw Food Fun for Families: Recipes and Tips for A Healthy Family Lifestyle,* will be available in 2014.

Karen travels throughout the United States and abroad delivering her impassioned message about raising healthy families. She is a staff writer for *Get Fresh*, *VegWorld* and *Vibrance* magazines. Karen is Health Expert Advisor for SAFbaby.com and has been a featured guest on numerous TV and radio talk shows.

Karen is also a speech pathologist and has been working with children for over 30 years, specialising in helping autistic children for the past 12 years. She incorporates health coaching into her programme and has seen significant progress in the children's communication skills and ability to focus and learn.

www.superhealthychildren.com

Nomi Shannon

Nomi Shannon is an award-winning author and world-renowned coach based in California in the USA. Her best-selling book, *The Raw Gourmet*, has sold over 150,000 copies. Her second book, *Raw Food Celebrations* (with S Duruz), is flying off the shelves at bookstores worldwide.

In 2008 Nomi received three Best of Raw Awards for Best Raw Educator, Favorite Raw Chef and Favorite Raw Book. In the 2009 and 2010 Best of Raw Awards, Nomi was placed in the top five in many categories including: Best Educator, Chef, Blog, Online Store and her personal favourite, Funniest Raw Woman.

A certified Hippocrates Health Educator and living foods vegan since 1987, Nomi has been featured in *Alive* magazine, *Get Fresh*, *San Diego North County Times* and *Galveston News*, as well as numerous radio shows and other media.

www.rawgourmet.com

Acknowledgements

There are so many people who contributed to this book, whether they realise it or not. Thanks are due to them all, but in particular: to Dr Colin McCarty, who planted the first seed; to Suzi McIntyre, who introduced me to far more than just dentistry; to Drs Brian and Anna Maria Clement and the Hippocrates Health Institute, for giving me access to so much more information and inspiration than I could have ever imagined; to my wonderful friends Rian, Trish, Amanda, Jo, Debbie and Dave – you know why; to my niece, Catherine, whose questions keep me on my toes; to my recipe contributors: Jessica, Nomi, Judy and Karen – your food is the best! To my fabulous partner Stewart, who has seen me through the late nights, the highs, the lows and everything in between, and who designed the cover; finally, to my parents, who supported me in my decision to study the sciences, and gave me the confidence to follow my dream. Arthur, my father, you didn't live to see this book published, but I hope I made you proud nonetheless.

Foreword

You have in your hands an invaluable guide to your body and to the most effective steps you can take so that it will function at its peak.

It's something few of us give much thought to, but it is only when our body is functioning at a high level that we are able to manifest our full potential in any area of life. None of us will show up as our most glorious self if our digestion is poor, our immune system under par, our blood sugar on a rollercoaster, or our brain chemistry out of whack. Yet so many of us go through life with all of these problems, and more – I certainly did for years. It is no surprise that all of these common problems so often manifest in unison, as they all have the same underlying cause – poor nutrition.

This book tells you how to eat for optimum health and if you follow the recommendations in it, chances are you will soon be feeling really rather fantastic. Follow them consistently and long term and you will reduce your risk of every single chronic illness from diabetes to depression to heart disease to cancer to dementia. You will also quickly start to lose any excess weight and to look your very best.

Perhaps vanity is a bigger motivator for you than either health or longevity. This was certainly true for me when I first became interested in nutrition as a teenager. It wasn't preoccupation with the health of my cells that was spurring me on in my quest for knowledge, but rather with the condition of my skin and the size of my thighs. Whatever your reason for wanting to learn more about nutrition, you've picked up the right book. In it, Max Tuck, aka the Raw Food Scientist, takes you on a tour of your body's nine systems – the digestive system, intestinal system, circulatory system, nervous system, immune system, respiratory system, urinary system, glandular system and structural system. She briefly outlines the physical structures of each system and their main functions, and follows this with advice about what you can eat, and otherwise do, to support each system.

If you already know a thing or two about nutrition you won't be surprised to read that the recommended foods are all nutrient-dense natural plant foods. These are the foods we should all be basing our diets around. As well as being the fuel the body needs to build healthy cells, they are also loaded with phytonutrients – bioactive compounds which actively protect against specific diseases and conditions. Plant foods are nature's medicines, but unlike pharmaceutical drugs, these medicines have no downsides.

Pharmaceutical drugs merely mask unwanted symptoms. They do nothing to address or eliminate the root cause of those symptoms. They are all, without exception, toxic to the body, and in all cases, the desired effect in the body comes at the expense of numerous undesired ones. This is why people who start taking one powerful drug so often soon develop a new condition for which they seek medical treatment, only to be prescribed a new drug to mask the symptoms of that, too – and on it goes. Contrast this with the healing power of natural plant foods. While a certain vegetable, herb or berry might have the greatest (known) benefits for, say, the circulatory system, it will always be beneficial for the other eight systems too. That is why the diet that most effectively lowers your cancer risk does just the same for your risk of heart disease, diabetes, depression and dementia, *and* will also slow the aging process and make your skin glow.

The reverse is true too. A food that is bad for one system of the body is bad for all systems. Let's take refined sugar as an example. We all know that refined sugar is a leading cause of tooth decay, but that's just the tip of the iceberg. Few realise that sugar also ages our skin, hardens our arteries, lowers our immunity, sends our hormones out of whack, damages our liver, brain and all of our other organs, and wreaks havoc with every system of the body.

Max Tuck's prescription for optimum health is as simple as it is sound: base your diet around whole, natural, raw, unprocessed plant foods; avoid manmade chemicals wherever possible; make exercise a part of your routine; cultivate a positive mental attitude; get plenty of fresh air and sunshine. She has been doing all of the above for two decades and is a shining example of what is possible for you, too, if you choose to follow her advice.

In 1990 Max was classified as a medical write-off due to her debilitating chronic fatigue. Doctors told her there was nothing that could be done – that her life would be compromised due to her condition, and that she would sadly never recover. Unwilling to accept this prognosis Max began researching health and nutrition. As she studied, gained insights and uncovered answers, she upgraded her food choices and her lifestyle, and within six months she had regained her health.

Today, far from leading a compromised life, Max has two careers – she is a veterinary surgeon as well as a health educator and author – and in her spare time competes in marathons, tri-athlons and other endurance events, climbs mountains, and has also gained a black belt in karate. By 1998 she had adopted the raw and living foods diet she still follows to this day. In chapter 1, Max outlines exactly what this way of eating entails, and why it brings health and longevity benefits like no other.

I know a thing or two about this topic as my own health quest brought the raw and living foods diet onto my radar in a big way 11 years ago. It was the summer of 2002, I was a new mum and I was at my local Planet Organic store in West London. I was looking for a healthy vegan cookbook but with every title I picked up, I found myself thumbing through recipes full of white flour, white sugar, margarine and/or heated oils. Then another book caught my eye. It had one word on the cover: RAW. As I picked it up and started reading about the health benefits of raw and living foods, a light bulb went on. I *knew*. I bought the book and immediately started following a very high-raw diet. I also read everything I could get my hands on and attended every seminar and lecture I could.

I later spent five years as the editor of a raw foods magazine, and now write a blog about achieving optimum health through a nutrient-dense high-raw diet. I continue to read every major book that is published on this topic, and I can tell you this: never before has a book about this way of eating better explained the specific effects of our diet and lifestyle choices on the body's organs and systems.

This book is the culmination of Max's scientific training, her personal determination to achieve optimum health, and her 23 years of dedicated study and practice towards not only achieving that goal, but continually expanding her knowledge and expertise. I wish it had been around when I started out on my own health quest. It would have saved me years of trial and error.

This compelling, no-nonsense and highly readable guide can turn your health, and your life, around. Enjoy the read, and the amazing benefits.

Sarah Best
www.sarahbesthealth.com

Preface

In October 1975, an enthusiastic young chemistry teacher stood up on stage in the assembly hall of a somewhat ordinary high school, situated on a small island off the south coast of England. He began by setting off explosions and mixing things in test tubes that gave off lots of coloured smoke. Sitting mesmerised in the audience was a 12-year-old girl with long blonde hair and a remarkable memory, who possessed a talent for languages and creative writing rather than science and maths. In that moment she knew that instead of wanting to follow a career that involved her hitherto passion for language, she would study science and find out what made those things explode and why the smoke was all sorts of different colours. Her parents knew better than to try to persuade her otherwise; this was one determined daughter that they had brought into the world.

That was my first introduction to Dr Colin McCarty, or 'The Doc' as he later became known. He was my high-school science teacher and the inspiration behind my choice of subjects to study. It fell to my older sister to suggest veterinary medicine; all I knew was that my career now had to involve science in some form, and in particular chemistry.

From that time forward, I found it increasingly difficult just to blindly accept what people told me was the truth. I always had to have proof, and there had to be solid evidence to support it. I did not consider myself to be a hardened sceptic; I just needed to know *why*.

It has been stated many times that scientific studies are fundamentally flawed, because just the act of observation can be sufficient to alter the outcome. However, the randomised, double blind, placebo-controlled crossover trial still remains the best tool that we have to minimise this inherent difficulty, and it is what the best experiments and studies consist of in modern scientific research. This can present difficulties if we want to study healthy populations and compare them with unhealthy ones, particularly in relation to their diets, since epidemiological studies are what we have to rely on in these instances. However, these can in their own right be of incredible value; take, for example, the well-known China Study by the highly respected author Dr T. Colin Campbell. Even this remarkable work has come up against staunch criticism, but I still firmly believe that many of the conclusions therein are inescapable: healthy diet = less degenerative disease, bad diet = more degenerative disease. Or, if you are a computer user, the well-known acronym GIGO – garbage in, garbage out.

When I think about food, and how it affects our bodies, I want to know exactly how it does it. What is going on biochemically? What are the different 'coloured-smoke equivalents' and how do they benefit us or harm us? When I first decided, or, should I say, was persuaded, to write this book, I wanted to take a systematic approach – after all, modern-day medicine is often taught on a systems basis. I even gave the book a working title of *The Nine Body Systems* whilst I was researching and writing it. What became immediately apparent, however, was the massive crossover between the various systems, which I hope you will find when you read what follows.

Whilst I have fundamentally written this book from the

perspective of a living foods lifestyle (which I personally follow), I have been keen to ensure that the information presented here is accessible to everyone, regardless of their current diet, since I believe that upgrades can always be made. From the awed 12-year-old to the vet who later became a health educator for people, my fascination with the power of food as medicine remains undimmed. I hope that you, too, will find inspiration in these pages.

Max Tuck, The Raw Food Scientist
2014

Chapter 1

What constitutes a healthy diet?

Let's get straight to the point: I recommend a plant-based diet. There are many reasons for this. I could go on about comparative anatomy and that we, as primates, have the dullest canine teeth of all, making them inappropriate and useless for meat-eating. However, having had to endure a lecture at university on the dentition of the Pleiocene giraffe, of all things, I will not bore you with such details. Instead I will focus on the benefits that the plant kingdom gives us, and the potential challenges we might face if we choose to base our diet on animal-derived products.

Don't get me wrong – I was brought up in a family that believed that the diet should be based upon meat and potatoes, with a few vegetables thrown in. Indeed, as a child, if I wasn't particularly hungry at any given mealtime, I was always encouraged to 'eat the meat and leave the rest'. When I chose to eliminate dairy products at the age of 15, as a result of my self-diagnosed dairy allergy, my parents were initially concerned about my protein intake and my bone strength, due to widely accepted dogma. Little did I know at the time that I was doing my bones a massive long-term favour.

I have no doubt that the debate as to whether humans are omnivorous, carnivorous or frugivorous (fruit and leaf eaters) will run and run. My approach to what to eat for optimal health is based upon the current available science. In the future, who knows what we will discover? What is certain is that we continue to unveil, on an almost daily basis, nutrients in the plant kingdom that have massive benefits not only for maintenance of overall health, but for the prevention, and even reversal, of certain disease states.

Some alarming statistics

We are now facing the alarming fact that one in two of us will die from heart disease, which will be the cause of 23.3 million deaths annually worldwide by 2030; one in three of us will succumb to cancer; three million Canadians have chronic respiratory disease; 10 per cent of all those in the USA over the age of 20 have chronic kidney disease; one in 12 has an autoimmune disease, according to the Arizona Center for Advanced Medicine; and diabetes and obesity rates are soaring. Anything that we can do to strengthen our bodies against such disease processes will surely be welcomed. I believe, and science is proving, that the nutrients found in plants have a major part to play here.

Plant or animal?

Firstly, I would like to look at the plant-based versus animal-based approach to nutrition from a macronutrient perspective. Macronutrients are the bulk components of our food, and are measured in grams: we're talking protein, fat and carbohydrate. In the past, it was believed that we could only obtain all the essential amino acids, the building-blocks of our proteins, from animal products. I always remember being told in a school biology class in the 1970s that the best way for us to build our own bodily muscle was to eat something that was identical in structure to our muscles – implying cannibalism. Since the laws of the land at that time prevented such activity (and, thankfully, still do), our second-best option was therefore the muscles of pigs, since biologically they were considered to be the closest 'edible' species to ourselves. Whether this was just the teacher's personal opinion or whether it was grounded in some sort of solid science of the time I do not know.

Fortunately for us, times have moved on. Far from being considered to be an inferior type of protein, we now know that certain plants contain all the essential amino acids that we need on a daily basis, so all that we need to do is eat the correct type of plant. Wheatgrass juice, sunflower greens, blue-green algae, hemp seeds and sprouted brown rice contain a complete spectrum of amino acids, rendering animal consumption unnecessary for obtaining adequate protein. Previously it was thought that unless we ate a full spectrum of amino acids at every meal, we would run the risk of protein deficiency. This myth was popularised in the early 1970s in the book *Diet for a Small Planet* by Frances Moore Lappé, who recommended 'protein combining' to avoid problems associated with the so-called 'incomplete proteins' that the plant kingdom provided. The author later revised these recommendations in 1998, and subsequent research has confirmed the protein-combining theory to be incorrect.

Following in-depth study of protein metabolism in humans, and summarised in 1994 in the *American Journal of Clinical Nutrition*, in a paper entitled 'Plant proteins in relation to human protein and amino acid nutrition' (by V.R. Young and and P.L. Pellett), the myth was dispelled once and for all, but still persists in some unenlightened circles: my niece was recently told at running camp that she *could* be a vegan athlete, but she would have to pay attention to protein combining. We only have to look at the incredible athletic feats of people such as Brendan Brazier, former professional Ironman triathlete, and Scott Jurek, the world's greatest-ever ultramarathon runner, to realise that a vegan diet is in no way inferior for the development of athletic prowess. Even an otherwise excellent review in 2001 from the Nutrition Committee of the American Heart Association, warning about the dangers of high-protein diets, made the mistake of citing Lappé's book (St. Jeor S, Howard B, Prewitt E, 'Dietary Protein and Weight Reduction', *Circulation* 2001; 104: 1869-74). Indeed, research now indicates that the greater the consumption of animal protein, the greater the incidence of degenerative disease – notably heart disease and cancer. We know that it is not the protein itself that is the problem; just its source. References to this can be found not only in *The China Study*, by T. Colin Campbell (BenBella Books, 2005) but also many other medical texts.

The pathways via which animal protein consumption degrades our health are many and varied. Considering it in relation to heart disease, William Castelli, MD, director of the Framingham Heart Study (the longest-running clinical study in medical history), is quoted as saying of the heart disease epidemic, 'If Americans adopted a vegetarian diet, the whole thing would disappear.' From this, I would go further to state that dairy products can be just as detrimental to heart health, since they contain high levels of fat, cholesterol and protein. We know that cholesterol is not the only factor involved in heart disease, and in fact C-reactive protein (CRP) and homocysteine levels are now considered to be much more accurate determinants of cardiac risk. Indeed, those on a vegan diet as opposed to a vegetarian one fare better in parameters for heart health, and many research papers now indicate that vegetarianism is insufficient to protect against the major disease processes, and that it only prolongs life expectancy by a somewhat disappointing five years more than an omnivorous approach. Lacto-ovo vegetarianism is no longer the prescription for health that was once believed.

A major study published in February 2005 reconfirmed the link between animal products and heart problems. The study, which was published in the *American Journal of Epidemiology*, concluded that out of 29,000 participants, those who ate the most meat were also at the greatest risk for heart disease (Kelemen et al. *American Journal of Epidemiology* 2005: 161(3); 239-249). The researchers also reported that a high intake of protein from vegetable sources such as tofu, nuts, and beans lowers the risk of heart disease by 30 per cent. Dr Linda E Kelemen, the lead scientist of the study, stated: 'Not all proteins are equal' – while vegetable protein can help to keep our hearts healthy, eating animal protein can shorten life expectancy.

A long-term study conducted by Harvard Medical School over a period in excess of 20 years has more recently indicated that the consumption of red meat increases the risk of death from cancer and heart disease (Pan et al, *Archives of Internal Medicine*. 2012; 172(7): 555-63). Just by adding an extra portion of unprocessed red meat to your daily diet causes an increased risk of death from any cause by 13 per cent, of fatal cardiovascular disease by 18 per cent and mortality from cancer by 10 per cent, with the figures being higher if that meat is processed. Could it be that we are finally waking up to the realisation that a plant-based diet is not just for tree-hugging freaks, but the *only* sensible choice for anyone who is seeking a long life free from the shackles of disease?

Cancer is beginning to overtake heart disease as the most common cause of our demise, and in Canada it now ranks as the number one cause of mortality, having recently knocked heart disease off the top spot. A recent study, entitled 'Vegerarian diets and the incidence of cancer in a low-risk population', published in *Cancer Epidemiology, Biomarkers and Prevention* (2013; 22(2): 286-94 from researchers at Loma Linda University, California (Tantamango-Bartley et al), reported that vegans have lower rates of cancer than both meat-eaters and vegetarians. In this study, vegan women had 34 per cent lower incidence of female-specific cancers such as breast, cervical and ovarian. This was when compared with a group of healthy omnivores who ate substantially less meat than the general population (two servings a week or more), as well as after controlling for non-dietary factors such as smoking, alcohol and familial history of cancer.

Numerous other studies comparing cancer rates in those who choose not to eat animal products have reported similar findings. Some studies indicate that vegetarians have similar cancer rates to meat eaters in regard to certain types of cancer. This probably highlights the fact that the vegetarians in these studies consumed dairy products and eggs, although this is purely my personal assumption. As I have stated, vegetarianism is not enough. If we want to give ourselves the greatest degree of protection from degenerative disease, I believe we have to take it further.

Obesity levels in the developed world are skyrocketing. Comparing vegetarians to meat eaters, a Swedish study published in the June 2005 issue of the *American Journal of Clinical Nutrition*, and involving 55,459 middle-aged healthy women, concluded that the non-meat-eating women weighed significantly less than the meat eaters, and had a lower BMI (Body Mass Index – a method of determining ideal weight ranges). The study, entitled 'Risk of overweight and obesity among semi-vegetarian, lactovegetarian and vegan women' (*American Journal of Clinical Nutrition* 2005: 81 (6); 1267-1274) was not a weight-loss study, and 25 per cent of the non-meat-eaters were overweight, but this compared with 40 per cent of the meat-eaters; again, a statistically significant measurement. The researchers found that vegetarians were two-thirds less likely than meat-eaters to be obese.

In line with obesity, the incidence of **diabetes** is also reaching epidemic proportions. According to Diabetes UK, the incidence of diabetes has risen from 1.4 million in 1996 to 2.9 million, and is estimated to reach 4.0 million by 2025 in the UK population. Type 2 diabetes is a lifestyle disease that can be prevented and reversed through dietary means and exercise. Its many complications include blindness, and the need for limb amputation as a result of tissue necrosis due to the compromised blood circulation to the extremities that is a feature of the disease. It is also increasingly being associated with dementia (Dominguez et al in *Neurologia* 2013: S0213-4853 (13) 00: 155-152). Why, I wonder, would a change in diet and lifestyle be considered to be so drastic when there is so much at stake?

An article published in *Diabetes Care*, the Journal of the American Diabetic Association (Tonstad et al, 'Type of vegetarian diet, body weight, and prevalance of type 2 diabetes', *Diabetes Care* 2009; 32(5): 791-796), assessed the prevalence of type 2 diabetes in people following different types of vegetarian diets compared with that in non-vegetarians. The main finding was that vegan and lacto-ovo-vegetarian diets were associated with a nearly one-half reduction in risk of type 2 diabetes compared with the risk associated with non-vegetarian diets after adjustment for a number of socioeconomic and lifestyle factors, as well as low BMI, that are typically associated with vegetarianism. The study indicated that vegetarian diets may in part counteract the environmental forces leading to obesity and increased rates of type 2 diabetes, but interestingly, only vegan diets were associated with a BMI in the optimal range.

With such compelling evidence in the medical literature indicating that meat eating, and the consumption of animal products in general, is linked to many (largely preventable) disease processes, is there any evidence that we cannot get all of the nutrients we need from the plant kingdom, thus necessitating the consumption of animal products? The Weston A. Price Foundation would say an emphatic 'yes' to this question. I, however, beg to differ. Having read their summary of the nutrients that it is impossible to obtain from the plant kingdom, and performed my own analysis, I find a shortfall in their evidence. I disagree that cholesterol is an essential nutrient; we manufacture it in the liver, unless we happen to have an incredibly rare genetic disorder, or we are under three years old, which I suspect readers of this book will not be. We can obtain vitamin K2, essential for bone health, from natto, a fermented soya product. The important fatty acids necessary for brain development can be found in flax oil and blue-green algae.

The vitamin B12 debate is potentially problematic. However, many non-vegans have vitamin B12 levels which are sub-optimal. See chapter 5, 'The nervous system', for more information on this vital nutrient, and why health experts state that it is the one supplement that everyone, regardless of their current diet, should take.

I personally conclude that a vegan diet can supply all the nutrients we need in abundance, provided that it is done correctly, together with judicious whole-food supplementation (to counteract the inherent difficulty with the nutrient-depleted soil in which most of our food is grown). There is a vast difference between a 'junk' vegan diet, based on processed meat substitutes and other such non-animal-derived nonsense, and one that is based on whole, ripe, fresh, unprocessed, and largely uncooked, produce. That is the diet that I advocate. That is what the bulk of this book is about.

Just boring salads?

For those who do not understand the concept of eating food uncooked, it raises many questions. People continue to ask me questions such as, 'Is bread raw?' (it isn't), 'So you drink soya milk then?' (no, I don't), and 'Don't you get fed up with only eating boring salads?' If only they knew. Whilst I would love to invite everyone to dinner to dispel some myths, that's not really a practical option, so here is a list of the 'food groups' of the plant kingdom that offer us the most major nutritional benefits, and around which I recommend that your diet should largely be based.

- Ripe fresh fruits
- Vegetables (especially brightly coloured ones)
- Leafy greens (e.g. spinach, rocket, kale, chard, watercress)
- 'Tray' greens (sunflower, wheatgrass, pea greens)

- Sprouted small-leaf seeds (e.g. alfalfa, onion, cress, broccoli)
- Wild greens (e.g. dandelion)
- Herbs (e.g. parsley, coriander)
- Sprouted pulses and beans (e.g. lentils, mung beans, chick peas)
- Sprouted grains (e.g. buckwheat, quinoa, amaranth, teff)
- Seeds (e.g. chia, pumpkin, sunflower)
- Unroasted, unsalted nuts (e.g. almond, brazil, pistachio)
- Sea vegetables/seaweeds (e.g. nori, dulse, wakame)
- Mushrooms
- Edible flowers
- Algae
- Cold-pressed unrefined oils (e.g. olive, flax, hemp)
- Superfoods
- Nut and seed butters
- Spices

As you can see, there is a lot of variety here, and whilst it may appear to be a far cry from a standard diet that we may have been brought up on, there are plenty of reasons for these recommendations: not just from the standpoint of them not containing elements that cause harm (animal protein, animal fat, etc) but because they contain substances, known to most scientists as phytonutrients (plant nutrients), that do us a whole power of good. Let's take a look at the list.

Ripe fruit and fresh vegetables contain a vast array of vitamins and antioxidants. In his book *Food IS Medicine, The Scientific Evidence*, Dr Brian Clement lists references to hundreds of scientific papers which indicate not only the general health benefits of such phytonutrients in these foods, for conditions ranging from allergies and arthritis to periodontal disease and stroke, but also evidence for the healing effects of nutrient synergies, and nutrient retention and health benefits of raw versus cooked/

processed vegetables. It's not exactly bedtime reading, but I'd say the book is a must for anyone interested in the science behind the nutritional benefits that the plant kingdom offers us.

Many of the known health benefits of eating brightly coloured plants come from the mineral and antioxidant levels found in these foods. Antioxidant content is specifically relevant, since the **oxidative stress theory** has now been proven beyond reasonable doubt to be the major cause of ageing and degenerative disease. The basis of this theory is that oxidative damage to cells increases with age, and that a state of chronic oxidative stress exists in all aerobic cells under normal metabolic conditions, as a result of an imbalance between pro-oxidants and antioxidants. The accumulation of oxidative damage leads to a progressive decline in the function of cellular processes. People who have higher blood levels of specific antioxidants have better protection from all causes of death, and the greater the spectrum of antioxidants, the greater the benefits.

We are finding more and more that we literally do need to 'eat the rainbow' to access the 25,000 or so different antioxidants that we so far know about, that are present in plants. I elaborate more on this subject in my CD *Oxidative Stress and the Link between Diet and Health*, but fundamentally, no one single colour of fruit, vegetable or berry contains all of the antioxidants that we need. We must eat red plants, yellow plants, green plants, orange plants, purple and blue plants, to access all of these amazing benefits. In orange plants alone, over 40 different types of carotenoid antioxidant have been discovered. In green plants, indole carbinols, isothiocyanates and sulforaphane, for example, have been demonstrated to have antioestrogenic properties, to prevent carcinogens from binding to DNA, and to reverse tumour development. That's just three phytonutrients. Imagine what benefits all 25,000, plus the many others that we are yet to discover, could have in our bodies, where it is stated that each one of our 50 trillion cells takes up to 10,000 oxidative 'hits' per day?

The benefits of plants do not end there. In the protein- and fat-dominant nuts and seeds, for example, we find essential fats that can help us to lower our blood cholesterol, improve the quality of our skin and help our brain perform at its optimal level. The minerals found in seaweeds help us to maintain our bone health and our thyroid health. The simple sugars that abound in fresh fruit enable us to fuel intense exercise. The fibre that is present in all plants brings about normal peristalsis (muscular contraction) of the bowel, eliminating constipation and reducing our risk of bowel cancer and elevated blood cholesterol. And that's just for starters.

With all of the known benefits that the plant kingdom gives us, I believe it is time fully to embrace a plant-based diet for our long-term health. After all, we don't just want to survive in our modern society – we deserve to thrive. I firmly believe that this lifestyle will allow us to do so in magnificent fashion.

Chapter 2

The digestive system

27 to 30 feet of gut, 1.7 litres of saliva per day, 500 kg of food per year – that's a lot of processing!

The digestive system, beginning with the mouth and continuing via the stomach and small intestine, allows us to break food down into smaller and smaller components, ending up with molecules which we can absorb and utilise for the production of energy and cell renewal. Finally, it packages the residue for 'waste disposal' via the large intestine.

So many people in our society have compromised digestion, and these days it is almost considered to be normal that people over the age of 40 have digestive difficulty. It absolutely does not have to be this way. The digestive system is very much more than just a length of gut. It also consists of digestive organs and glands, and by understanding how these function, we can learn how to optimise our digestive capacity and feel amazing.

How frequently do we see TV ads for products that 'help' with indigestion? In fact, they don't help us at all. All they do is reduce the pain we experience from eating in an inappropriate way, and do nothing actually to aid digestive function. More than that, they harm it, but we'll get onto that point a little later.

So, why is digestion important? It's a simple enough question, but have you ever stopped to consider exactly what that length of gut is doing for you? Fundamentally, it is allowing us to access the nutrients in our food, so that we can build a strong, healthy body. Therefore, since we already know that we are not just what we eat (we are what we eat, digest, absorb, utilise and fail to eliminate), that 27 feet of gut and its associated organs and glands are either ensuring you make the best use of the food you are eating or not. After all, what is the point in eating excellent food if you can't access the valuable nutrition that it contains? You might as well just flush it down the toilet and cut out the middle man...

Meet your digestive system

Your digestive system (gastrointestinal or 'GI tract') consists anatomically of:

Teeth
Mouth
Oesophagus
Stomach (cardiac and pyloric parts)
Duodenum (upper small intestine)
Jejunum (middle small intestine)
Ileum (lower small intestine)
Caecum (junction of small and large intestine)
Ascending colon (large intestine)
Transverse colon (large intestine)
Descending colon (large intestine)
Rectum
Anus

The glands and other structures associated with it are:
Salivary glands
Liver and gall bladder
Pancreas
Lymphatics

The most obvious signs of poor digestion are a feeling of bloatedness, or excess gas/belching after meals, or discomfort or heartburn after eating certain types of food. Many people complain, as they get older, of not being able to digest everything they could when they were younger. However, some other signs of poor digestion might not be quite so immediately recognisable, despite having their roots in the digestive system. These include symptoms as diverse as general weakness or lethargy, body odour or bad breath, food allergies, skin problems, headaches and even weak fingernails.

Despite the numerous glands and structures associated with the digestive system, and the potentially complex interrelationship between them, there are a number of straightforward ways in which digestion can be improved, so don't panic! Let's start right at the top – in the mouth.

A very simple way immediately to improve digestion is by more thoroughly chewing the food. This will allow more time for salivary amylase, a starch-digesting enzyme, to be mixed with the food and therefore start the process of digestion. An old Indian saying is 'Chew your food, because your stomach has no teeth.' Digestion is kick-started in the mouth, and it's really no surprise that people who eat very fast without proper chewing often end up with the pain associated with indigestion. Chew your food until it begins to turn liquid.

Not everyone is able to chew their food thoroughly. For those with dental difficulties, endless chewing may be an option they are unable to tolerate. In these cases blending is helpful, also being useful for anyone who generally suffers poor digestion. Ann Wigmore, the original founder of the Hippocrates Health Institute, was a great believer in the power of blending and its health benefits. Although a few nutrients (such as very sensitive phytonutrients and enzymes) will be damaged by blending as a result of oxidation, the majority will be made more accessible because the cell walls of the plants will be broken down. You will

14

therefore have to spend less of your energy on digestion, freeing it up for other functions, such as building new cells, kicking out infections, healing, running your metabolism and detoxification. Blended soups and smoothies are a great way to maximise nutrition without stressing the digestive system, provided that the principles of good food combining are followed.

What's all this about food combining?

The Hay diet was the first diet, as I recall, which popularised the concept of food combining to improve digestive health and alleviate certain medical conditions. However, the initial concept can be traced back further to Pavlov, the Russian scientist more famous for his work with dogs. It used to be thought that if food was eaten raw, correct food combining was irrelevant, since the live enzymes in the food itself were not destroyed by cooking and could therefore break the food down, but we now know otherwise. An optimally combined raw food meal will give you improved digestion and therefore greater assimilation of the nutrients present.

The fundamental principles of food combining are to keep proteins away from starches, and eat fruit on its own if you are having it. Having fruit as a dessert, for example, is unfortunately very bad for the digestive function. I recommend having protein-rich foods earlier in the day, since they take up to four hours to digest, and require an acidic digestion. Carbohydrate (starch-based) foods generally require alkaline digestion and take up to three hours to digest, so they are better as an evening meal. In simplistic terms, if we try to digest foods that require acidic digestion together with those that require alkaline digestion in the same meal, it is the equivalent of throwing everything in the washing machine at the same time and not separating your whites from your delicates. Neither fabric gets its ideal treatment.

Below are some of the food group options to be aware of in regard to living foods. Please also see the food combining chart on page 17 for further clarification.

1. Proteins: Digestion time four hours
    Seeds, such as pumpkin, sesame, hemp and sunflower. Nuts, such as almonds, Brazil nuts, pecans, pine nuts, walnuts.

2. Starches: Digestion time three hours
    Sprouted grains, such as amaranth, quinoa, millet, rye. Sprouted legumes, such as chickpeas and lentils. Winter squashes, sweet potatoes and yams.

3. Vegetables: Digestion time two and a half hours
    Sprouted small-leaf greens, such as alfalfa, radish, clover. Fruit-vegetables, such as cucumber, red pepper, summer squash, courgette. Leafy greens, such as rocket, spinach, chard, watercress, cabbage, kale. Low starch root vegetables, such as carrots, parsnips, beets and radishes.

4. Fruits: Digestion time two hours (15 to 30 minutes for melons)
    Acid fruits, such as grapefruit and orange. Sub-acid fruits, such as apples, apricots, berries, grapes, mango and peach. Sweet fruit, such as all dried fruit, bananas, persimmons.

Good live-food combination examples would include, for example:

- Avocado and greens
- Avocado and sub-acid fruit
- Protein and sprouts and leafy greens
- Starch and sprouts and vegetables

Poor combinations would be:

- Fruit and starch
- Fruit and vegetable
- Fruit and protein

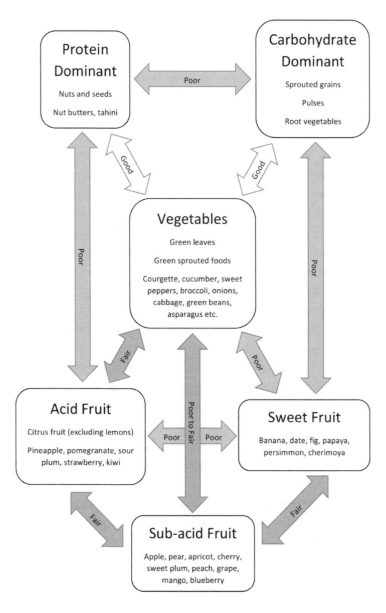

All melons should be eaten alone.
Avocados are best combined with acid or sub-acid fruits or green vegetables.
Each group only contains a selection of the common foods available.

Figure 1: Food Combining Chart

- Starch and protein
- Starch and avocado

In addition to considering the benefits of good food combining to aid the digestive function, fermenting is also a great way to break down the tough plant cellulose (a structural component of the cell walls of plants) to make it more digestible. I have to say at this point, not everyone likes fermented food. I personally can't stand it and never eat it. However, it is very good from a digestive perspective and if you don't mind the smell and taste of vinegar, you'll find that fermented foods such as home-made sauerkraut and kimchee could be your best friends at lunchtime. Fermented food is great not just from the perspective of being easy to digest and nutritious, but also because of the extra probiotics (friendly bacteria) that you'll access from it (see chapter 3, page 44).

Many people find that they experience bloating and gas when they first commence a living foods regime. This is often as a result of poor digestive function, and can be easily alleviated by taking digestive enzymes with each meal, either in capsule form with water directly before eating, or by sprinkling the capsule contents onto your food. I recommend the use of HHIZyme (see page xxx), made by the Hippocrates Institute.

Altogether, up to 75 per cent of the energy used by the body is used in the digestion of cooked food, particularly if that food is calorie- and sugar-laden, poorly assimilable and lacking in essential nutrients. Further information on this subject can be found in *Life Force – Superior Health and Longevity* by Dr Brian Clement, PhD (Healthy Living Publications, 2007). Nutrient-rich, easily digested food can be assimilated with less energy expenditure, so by eating food ripe, raw, enzymatically intact and properly combined to alleviate digestive stress, you can free up a huge amount of energy to be used in whatever way you want – that is, for exercise, hobbies and so on. We all know that 'fall asleep in the afternoon' feeling after traditional Christmas dinner, don't we? That's because all our energy is going towards digestion and there isn't enough to keep us awake.

I also recommend juices for top-quality nutrition, since they require minimal digestion. Green juices are perfect because they contain high-quality, bioavailable protein which is immediately available for absorption with no effort required. We want our proteins as individual amino acids, and I recommend that since meat and animal protein generally are very difficult to digest, and give a wide range of other problems, they are best avoided.

My daily green juice

As mentioned above, the best type of juice is the green juice. This may vary in its list of ingredients, but always has a base of cucumber and celery, with sunflower green sprouts and pea shoots. Here's why I recommend this combination of ingredients. Cucumber is a great base since it is a non-sweet fruit and is very hydrating. During our busy lives it is essential to remain hydrated. Celery adds minerals and gives a slightly salty taste that most people find very pleasant. It is also a good source of organic sodium, a mineral that many people are deficient in, particularly those with adrenal exhaustion (I explain this on page 127) or anyone suffering from chronic stress. If you happen to be a celery hater you can just use less of it, or omit it completely, but then you'll miss out on some of the benefits. If you use only a little in a large juice you'll probably not even notice that it's there.

Sunflower greens are very high in protein and contain a complete spectrum of essential amino acids. Protein in the juice helps to balance blood sugar and eliminate the risk of cravings. For those interested in energy systems and, in particular, Kirlian photography (an ultraviolet film technique considered to give an indication of the bioelectricity, and therefore 'life force' of objects), it's fascinating to see that the sunflower green sprout has a Kirlian field that extends out two feet (61cm) in every direction, making it the most energetic of all plants. Dr Valerie Hunt of the Bioenergy Fields Foundation of California has used Kirlian photography to carefully document her findings about the bioelectricity of cells. In addition to having a large Kirlian field, sunflower greens are a fantastic source of enzymes and chlorophyll. Pea shoots are also an excellent and balanced source of protein and give a slightly sweet taste to the juice. Personally I feel it is essential to use sprouts in the green drinks, since they contain 10 to 30 times the nutritional value of the best-quality standard vegetables. Avoid them and your cells won't be as well fed as they deserve.

The above ingredients are the standard **Hippocrates Green Drink**, which is served three times daily at the Hippocrates Health Institute in Florida, the centre at which I received my live-food nutritional training, and also used on all fasting days. The reason is simple. It is highly digestible, provides a full spectrum of macro- and micro-nutrients, is rich in minerals and provides rapid hydration , whilst also avoiding any insulin surges.

So in summary, our easy-to-digest juice consists of:
- Celery
- Cucumber
- Sunflower greens
- Pea shoots

But now comes the fun part. We can make additions, depending on what we fancy. Personally I never tire of the above list, but do quite frequently add extras, such as:
- Kale: adds extra protein and minerals
- Lemon: adds alkalising minerals and gives a tang to the juice
- Lime: for the same reasons as lemon above
- Garlic: fantastic for general detoxification and great for the immune system

- Ginger: anti-inflammatory, warming and has benefits for the circulation
- Liquid blue-green algae: for extra enzymes, minerals, chlorophyll, brain-boosting properties, mood stabilisation, alkalisation and avoidance of cravings. This creates a real superjuice, and in my opinion is an absolute must for anyone with blood sugar regulation issues or mood swings.
- Wheatgrass juice: ideally taken on an empty stomach half an hour before other liquids. If you can't handle the unusual taste it can be added to the green drink. Wheatgrass juice is a highly concentrated source of chlorophyll and contains 102 vitamins and minerals. It has a host of other benefits, which you can read all about on my website www.therawfoodscientist.com

A further recommendation that helps to improve digestive 'fire', which I learned from Viktoras Kulvinskas, co-founder of the Hippocrates Health Institute, whilst I was studying there, is as follows:

On rising, drink half a pint of water to which has been added the juice of 1 lemon and a pinch of cayenne pepper. The cayenne stimulates the secretion of hydrochloric acid which is important for protein digestion, and has a secondary benefit of improving the circulation (important if your circulatory function is poor). The lemon juice, despite containing citric acid, is actually alkalising to the body as a result of its mineral content, and will help to flush the kidneys. Those who do this every day will usually see great benefits within a month.

Low hydrochloric acid?

Amongst natural health practitioners, a recognised condition which could be affecting your digestive system is **hypochlorhydria**, which is basically less hydrochloric acid (HCl) in the stomach than we actually require . We need adequate HCl for the following reasons:

- Absorption of the following essential nutrients is dependent on adequate stomach acid: calcium, vitamins B9 and B12, magnesium, zinc, iron, vitamin C, and beta carotene. Having low HCl levels affects the absorption of the antioxidant vitamins A and E, putting you at greater risk of oxidative stress and chronic inflammation.
- Breakdown and initial digestion of protein for use in tissue and muscle synthesis.
- Activation of enzymes, hormones, and neurotransmitters.
- Prevention of bacterial pathogens from going into the lower GI tract. If pathogens are not destroyed, they can potentially put you at risk of disease and stomach cancer.

A common misconception is that Westerners have too much stomach acid – after all, antacids are incredibly popular – but this is rarely true. A more common problem is having much too little stomach acid for appropriate digestion, which produces gastric stress and can greatly increase your risk of stomach cancer. A serious but common problem is that because low stomach acid leads to impaired digestion, it is often misdiagnosed as there being too much stomach acid. This is because when the stomach does not empty correctly, partly digested carbohydrates and proteins that have started to ferment in the stomach will back up into the oesophagus, giving a burning sensation ('acid reflux') – an uncomfortable problem that is interpreted by many as resulting from excessive stomach acid.

One research study indicated that people with hypochlorhydria tended to experience much more acid reflux when lying down than those with normal stomach acid. Over half of these people had previously been misdiagnosed by a doctor as having too much stomach acid, and had been told to take antacids. This mis-diagnosis and subsequent use of antacids then puts the patient at risk for chronic disorders such as bone fractures and osteoporosis because important minerals, such as calcium and magnesium, and essential vitamins, such as vitamin K, are not being adequately absorbed. I discuss this issue more in my book *Top 10 Raw Food Tips for Osteoporosis*, but suffice it to say that bone fracture rates triple in individuals with low stomach HCl.

There are tests which can be performed to check whether or not you have adequate levels of hydrochloric acid in your stomach. The Heidelberg pH test is probably the most accurate way to gauge HCl insufficiency. However, this test is invasive and hospitals providing this service may not be easy to find. Hair tissue mineral analysis seems to correlate well with the Heidelberg test, and this test is more widely available. Dr John McLaren-Howard, from the specialist UK research laboratory Acumen, proposes a third option, a salivary VEGF (vascular endothelial growth factor) test. Most research on VEGF relates to high levels, but the opposite is also true, and low levels indicate hypochlorhydria. If you have been diagnosed with poor digestive function, it's a good idea to take one of the above tests for low HCl. Beware of the 'do it yourself at home' test involving betaine hydrochloride capsules. Not only is this test considered by experts to be highly inaccurate, it could also be dangerous, since it can increase the risk of gastric ulceration.

If your gastric HCl levels prove to be inadequate, supplemen-tation with oral HCl is a recommended approach. However, if you have, or are at risk from, gastric ulceration, you should not be taking supplemental HCl without following medical advice. Dr Gabriel Cousens, Director of the Tree of Life Rejuvenation Centre in Arizona, states that 50 per cent of people over the age of 60, and 80 per cent of those over the age of 85, have digestive problems caused by low gastric HCl. He recommends betaine hydrochloride, made from beetroot, as the best supplement for increasing your HCl levels and to enhance digestive function.

Dental problems?

There are many people who have dental trouble, and the health of the mouth is often considered to be a reflection of the health of the rest of the body. How many are aware, for example, that some of the organisms which are present in an unhealthy mouth can also be found in the heart, liver and kidneys? Degenerative disease affecting the heart valves may well have had its beginnings in a less than healthy mouth; certainly this is known to be a cause of heart disease in dogs, and human research is indicating the same thing. Dental health is often overlooked as a concept in whole body health, but it is an important factor nonetheless. For example, there are known links between health disorders, particularly affecting the nervous system, and mercury fillings; mercury is the most toxic metal that we can be exposed to. Additionally there is a suspected link between root canal treatments and breast cancer; a German study published approximately 10 years ago indicated that of 68,000 women who had received root canal treatments, 62 per cent had breast cancer on the side that related to the root canal treatment. A Japanese study indicated an even higher correlation. Put in these terms, looking after one's teeth takes on a somewhat more important health angle.

A concern for many people who are just commencing a raw food diet is that their dental health can deteriorate. This is definitely a problem in those who consume a large quantity of fruit, since the fruit sugar can damage the enamel over time, causing it to thin and the teeth to become sensitive. I personally fell into this trap initially. I understand that it is more of a concern in people who do not have access to ripe tropical fruit – that is, those who live in northern Europe or northern states of the USA or Canada. To avoid spoilage, fruit that is to be shipped over long distances is picked before it is fully ripe, and therefore it tends to be acid-forming. If in the tropics, I believe it is fine to eat the fruit there, but for those who live further north a high unripe, or artificially ripened, fruit intake can lead to dental decay. It was only when I switched to a diet based on dark green leaves, and drastically reduced my fruit intake, that my teeth actually stopped hurting.

Oral health can be improved by careful attention to both brushing and flossing. Removal of plaque is essential for reducing the incidence of gum disease, but, unlike many dentists, I do not recommend the use of fluoride in toothpaste, or drinking water for that matter. Fluoride is a by-product of the agricultural ferti-liser industry. It is a powerful toxic agent that was used during the holocaust to render prisoners sterile, and very effective it was too. It weakens bones and has adverse effects on the central nervous system. Do your own research as well, rather than just taking my word for it, but seek out an alternative to this destructive poison. In addition to brushing with fluoride-free toothpastes, chewing wheatgrass blades is helpful for the improvement of gum disease, as are natural mouthwashes that contain myrrh.

No discussion on the digestive system would be complete without considering digestive enzyme supplementation. Digestive enzymes are a staple of the Hippocrates programme, and for anyone with poor digestion or medical conditions such as irritable bowel syndrome (IBS) or Crohn's Disease, they are, in my opinion, essential. They contain the enzymes needed for splitting protein, carbohydrate and fats down into their component parts and enable us to access much more of the beneficial nutrition in the plants that we are eating, reducing digestive stress in the process. I have already mentioned the capsules that I recommend for this; they are called HHI-Zyme and are available via the Hippocrates Health Institute shop, or from Antidote for Modern Living in the UK (see the resources section at the end of the book).

Finally, I suggest you should try resting your digestive system by practising intermittent fasting. This is widely gaining acceptance and being validated scientifically for its many potential physiological benefits. You can read more about this in chapter 11.

The liver

A 1.5 kg miracle

Ah, the liver, that most abused organ. The liver is your largest internal organ and it performs an amazing array of tasks that I'll bet you didn't even realise. Here's a list of just a few of them:
- processing digested food from the intestine
- controlling levels of fats, amino acids and glucose in the blood
- combatting infections in the body
- clearing the blood of particles and infections including bacteria
- neutralising and destroying drugs and toxins
- manufacturing bile
- storing iron, vitamins and other essential chemicals
- breaking down food and turning it into energy
- manufacturing, breaking down and regulating numerous hormones including sex hormones
- making enzymes and proteins which are responsible for most chemical reactions in the body, for example those involved in blood clotting and repair of damaged tissues.

We tend to think of the liver as just an organ of detoxification, which it is almost by default, but it does so much more than that. In fact, one of its most important functions, which is so often overlooked, is that of energy production. In every one of your liver cells, there is a power generator in the form of a process called the 'Krebs cycle', or 'citric acid cycle' as it is also known.

Whilst this cycle goes on in the mitochondria of every single one of your bodily cells (except red blood cells, which have no mitochondria), the number of mitochondria in the cells of each organ is variable, dependent on the amount of energy that organ produces and needs. The liver cells have one of the highest concentrations of mitochondria in the body (second only to muscle

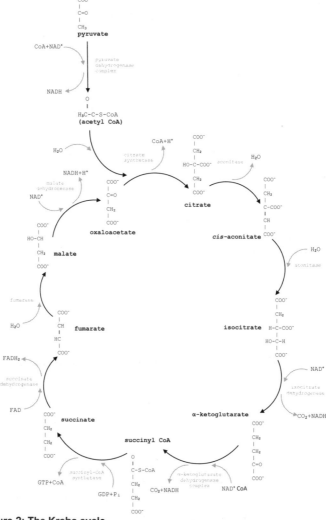

Figure 2: The Krebs cycle

cells), so now is an opportune time to talk about energy production. The multi-stage Krebs cycle allows glucose, from our food, to be turned into energy. If the liver isn't working too well, that could be the reason why you feel sluggish – not enough energy in the form of ATP (of which, more later on – see page 142) being generated.

Figure 2 is a diagram of the Krebs cycle. It's complicated, but so are your mitochondria, the organelles inside the cell where all this takes place. Some people still argue that it doesn't matter what you shove in at the top, because you still get energy out at the other end, but let's consider this for a moment: the Krebs cycle does not just run on glucose. It also requires oxygen, water and enzymes, and those enzymes require alkaline minerals for their production. Minerals, it could be stated, are the enzymes for the enzymes, so choose your fuel carefully. Let's consider the difference between trying to run the cycle on doughnuts and doing so on carrots or broccoli.

Stick a doughnut in the top of the Krebs cycle as a glucose source and what happens? Does the doughnut contain glucose? Yes. Loads of it, in fact. Water? No. Oxygen? No. Alkaline minerals? No. Enzymes? No. OK, what about carrots, or broccoli? Do they contain glucose? Yes. Water? Yes, of course, all fruits and vegetables contain organic water. Alkaline minerals? Yes. Enzymes? Yes, as long as you are having the vegetables in their raw state. Oxygen? Yes, potentially, especially if you are using the dark green leafy vegetables and tray greens, such as sunflower greens and pea shoots (which, according to Dr Brian Clement, in his books *LifeForce* and *Living Foods for Optimum Health* are a source of oxygen for the body), and you are juicing them. See the difference? If you are trying to make your Krebs cycle run on doughnuts, the body has to provide all the other factors that are needed to make it run, and that means a lot of input, which is metabolically draining. If on the other hand we use vegetables, raw or juiced, as our fuel source, many of the necessary elements are already present in the food, so the body has to do less work and use up fewer of its resources to make the cycle run. This is what is known as food that 'burns cleanly', and it's why I put all my athlete clients on fresh juices. I do, however, know some athletes who believe that it is perfectly adequate to fuel their activities with, for example, Christmas cake. These seem to be the athletes that are more injury prone and therefore have a lower 'life expectancy' in their sport. If you were an athlete (and perhaps you are), what would you rather have?

On now to other aspects of how important the liver is, and what can slow down its efficiency.

Bile production

Bile is interesting stuff. Greenish in colour, and fairly unpleasant-smelling, it is produced in the body of the liver, stored in the gall bladder and passes down the common bile duct into the small intestine. Its function is simple – it 'emulsifies' fats. Now we all know that oil and water don't mix, so bile allows the process of fat digestion to begin through this emulsification. Poor liver function often means reduced bile production and therefore diminished digestion, absorption and subsequent utilisation of essential fats.

We so often hear about gall bladder problems, and I know so many people who have had a cholecystectomy (gall bladder removal) performed, it seems almost as common as taking a bath! However, do bear in mind that every part of your anatomy is there for a reason, and we don't actually come into this world with any spare parts. This means that although we can actually survive without a gall bladder (or a spleen, or a right arm for that matter), we do better if we can keep it. One of the main reasons for performing this particular type of surgery is the presence of gall stones, which are made, fundamentally, from cholesterol. Since cholesterol is absent from all plants, it therefore perhaps stands to reason that you would only 'need' to have your gall bladder removed if you have gall stones from too much cholesterol in your system, in turn from eating animals and their derivatives.

For those who are concerned about any gall bladder sediment that may have been building up over the years, please see page 32 for how to conduct a liver and gall bladder flush. Do be aware that if you have already been diagnosed with gall stones, this procedure could potentially be dangerous for you, so take advice from your healthcare provider before proceeding with this one.

Alcohol

Any discussion on liver health would not be complete without a mention of that great liver-cell killer, alcohol. No matter how many studies have shown the damaging effects of alcohol consumption, there will always be some who still believe that red wine has benefits because of its antioxidant properties. Don't be fooled. Most of the so-called 'research' that supports this view has been funded by those with a vested interest, or is spouted by those who refuse to eliminate alcohol from their lives and so come up with some half-baked excuse that it somehow has health benefits. (Note, these are the people who are usually doing absolutely nothing else that would be remotely associated with health improvement.) Alcohol not only kills liver cells, it also disrupts the function of brain cells. Would you like to manage with fewer brain cells? Personally I want to keep my brain fully functional.

Alcohol breakdown in the liver is a brilliant example of the law of adaptive secretion of enzymes. Alcohol dehydrogenase (ADH) and aldehyde dehydrogenase (ALDH2) are the two enzymes that are your best friends if you choose to consume alcohol. And guess what? The more alcohol you drink, the more of these enzymes your liver will produce to help you to break down and eliminate this poison. Have you ever wondered why certain people who drink alcohol on a regular basis can go out on a Friday or Saturday night and drink 12 pints of beer and still be conscious? They are producing a stack of ADH and ALDH2, which is fundamentally keeping them alive, but at huge metabolic cost. It likewise explains why people who drink very little, or no alcohol at all, get drunk incredibly fast if they have alcohol even in small amounts – the liver only has to produce tiny quantities of these enzymes to deal with environmental ethanol that we might be exposed to, so a great stimulus is not there. I can't remember the last time I had alcohol, but I know exactly what would happen to me if I ever did.

So, if we produce these two enzymes in response to alcohol consumption and can therefore break alcohol down into, ultimately, carbon dioxide and water, what's the problem? The problem is a big one, and its name is acetaldehyde. Acetaldehyde is a highly toxic molecule and known carcinogen, which is produced early on in the breakdown of alcohol by the enzyme ADH. Chemically, acetaldehyde is similar to formaldehyde. By binding to certain proteins in the liver cells, acetaldehyde causes those cells to swell and malfunction, in addition to impairing the activity of certain enzymes. Acetaldehyde, either on its own or via other chemical binding reactions, favours the process of 'lipid peroxidation': a powerful pro-oxidant pathway, which, as we have learned above, contributes to the ageing process. Furthermore, the acetaldehyde-protein combination triggers an immune response which is thought to perpetuate alcohol-induced liver damage.

Acetaldehyde is known to cross the blood-brain barrier, and the brain is therefore not exempt from its toxic effects. In addition to disrupting the neurotransmitters, dopamine turnover increases, which in turn can have many detrimental effects, such as impairment of learning, impairment of spatial working memory and reduced visual discrimination.

Finally, alcohol consumption is implicated in the development of certain cancers, including those of the upper respiratory system, liver, colon and breast (Bagnardi et al, 'Alcohol consumption and the risk of cancer: a meta-analysis', *Alcohol Research & Health* 2001; 25(4): 263–270). Many of the toxic effects of alcohol consumption are attributable to acetaldehyde.

Protocol for liver and gall bladder flush

Many natural health practitioners recommend a liver cleanse, or 'liver flush', as a tool for detoxification. There are several protocols that you'll find on the internet, many of which, in my opinion, will be adding more toxins than they will be eliminating. Anna-Maria Clement, co-director of the Hippocrates Health Institute, suggests the following protocol as a safe and effective way of eliminating biliary 'sludge' and small gallstones.

This flush needs to be done over a period of five days. It is suitable for most people, but those who have been diagnosed with large gallstones would need to take medical advice before attempting it. Likewise, since it involves a short period of fasting, it is unsuitable for those who are underweight, pregnant or nursing mothers, children, or insulin-dependent diabetics. If you are in any doubt, always check with your healthcare professional prior to embarking on it. During the liver flush you may continue to take green juices and wheatgrass, but no food should be taken other than what is listed below for each day. You will need:

  Whole flax seeds (for flax water)
  Several bulbs of garlic
  Several organic apples
  Organic olive oil, in a dark glass bottle
  Several organic lemons
  A booking for colonic hydrotherapy on the morning of day 5.

Colonic hydrotherapy will maximise the detoxification process by removing impacted residue from the colonic wall, and aid in the elimination of any gallstones that have reached the large intestine. The liver flush will still be effective without it, but those who have sluggish liver function will also be likely to have accumulated waste in the colon, which in turn can attract the growth of anaerobic and 'unfriendly' bacteria, which feed off this waste. I therefore recommend having a colonic to eliminate this, for the best health-promotion benefits, and fastest elimination of waste products released by the liver and gallbladder flush.

Day 1

Drink some flax water (water that has had some flax seeds put in it and soaked overnight the night before). This is to protect the oesophagus and stomach from a possible burning sensation from the large amounts of garlic you will be taking in. The flax water can be used throughout the flush but you may find that it isn't needed after day 2. The flax water needs to be stored in the fridge.

Half an hour after drinking the flax water, start taking the garlic. To get the quantities of garlic that are needed, slice the garlic thinly and slice the apple thinly. Make a little 'sandwich' with apple on the outside and garlic as the filling. On day 1, take three cloves of garlic three times a day, with just enough apple to get the garlic down.

Garlic is an excellent food for detoxification, hence its use in the liver flush. It is antibacterial, antiparasitic and antiviral. Apples are used for their pectin content – apple pectin softens any cholesterol deposits in the liver and makes its passage through the biliary channels easier. Apple pectin has also been shown to lower blood LDL ('bad' cholesterol – Brouns et al, 'Cholesterol-lowering properties of different pectin types of mildly hypercholesterolemic men and women', *European Journal of Clinical Nutrition* 2012; 66(5): 591-599).

Day 2

As for day 1.

Day 3

Take four cloves of garlic three times a day with the apple. Just before bedtime, drink four fluid ounces of organic olive oil, followed immediately with four fluid ounces of freshly squeezed lemon juice. The olive oil stimulates the production of bile, and the lemon juice is sour/bitter, a combination which stimulates the flow of bile.

Day 4

Take five cloves of garlic three times a day with the apple. Again, just before bedtime, use the same amount of olive oil followed by lemon juice, as on day 3.

Day 5

In the morning, before eating anything or having green juice, have a colonic. You will pass anything up to 1500 small stones with the colonic if you have been on a standard Western diet. There are many practitioners of colonic hydrotherapy in developed countries, but when choosing your therapist it is best to go on recommendation. It is considered to be a safe practice, with the only contra-indications being those diagnosed with colon cancer or advanced Crohn's Disease.

Foods for liver health

What can you do today to help your liver, and therefore your digestive and immune systems, to work better? How about considering the following foods, which are great for liver health.

Garlic

Just a small amount of this pungent bulb has the ability to activate liver enzymes that helps your body flush out toxins. Garlic also holds high amounts of allicin and selenium, two natural compounds that aid in liver cleansing.

Grapefruit

High in both vitamin C and antioxidants, grapefruit increases the natural cleansing processes of the liver. A small glass of freshly squeezed grapefruit juice will help boost production of liver detoxification enzymes that help flush out carcinogens and other toxins. Naringenin, the main bioflavonoid in grapefruits, is more bioavailable when the fruit is juiced than when it is eaten whole.

Beetroot and carrot

Both extremely high in plant-flavonoids and beta-carotene, eating both beetroots and carrots can help stimulate and improve overall liver function.

Green tea

This interesting leaf is high in catechins, a plant antioxidant that is known to assist the liver's overall functions. Green tea has been the subject of a number of studies, which indicate that it has many positive effects, including the reduction of bad cholesterol, the inhibition of cancer cell growth and even protection against Alzheimer's disease. However, do be aware that green tea contains caffeine, which is an undesirable chemical compound. For those transitioning off coffee, however, green tea is a great alternative which has been shown to have various health benefits.

Green leafy vegetables, including wheatgrass juice

One of our most powerful allies in cleansing the liver, leafy greens are best eaten raw or juiced. Extremely high in plant chlorophylls, greens bind environmental toxins from the blood stream. With their distinct ability to neutralise heavy metal toxicity, chemicals and pesticides, these cleansing foods offer a powerful protective mechanism for the liver.

Try incorporating leafy greens such as bitter gourd, arugula, dandelion greens, spinach, mustard greens and chicory into your diet. This will help increase the creation and flow of bile, which in turn helps to remove waste from the organs and blood.

Avocados

This fatty fruit helps the body to produce glutathione, often called the 'master enzyme' of the body. Composed of the amino acids cysteine, glutamine and glycine, glutathione is concentrated in the liver, but also works throughout the body. This important enzyme is involved in protecting cells from environmental toxins, drugs and alcohol as well as toxins produced by the body itself as a result of normal metabolism. Studies presented in 2000 by Japanese researchers (American Chemical Society (2000, December 20). Avocados Contain Potent Liver Protectants. *ScienceDaily*. Retrieved November 5, 2013, from http://www.sciencedaily.com¬ /releases/2000/12/001219074822.htm) indicate the potential for improved liver health in humans when avocados are eaten regularly, if this study, conducted on rats, can be extrapolated to human health.

Apples

High in pectin, apples hold the chemical constituents needed for the body to cleanse and release toxins from the digestive tract. This, in turn, makes it easier for the liver to handle the toxic load during the cleansing process. Green apples, such as Granny Smith, contain the most pectin.

Olive oil and other oils

Cold-pressed organic oils such as olive, hemp and flax-seed are great for the liver, when used unheated, such as in salad dressings. Olive oil, in particular, has been demonstrated in the laboratory to reduce oxidative stress (Nakbi et al, 'Effects of olive oil and its fractions on oxidative stress and the liver's fatty acid composition in 2,4-Dichlorophenoxyacetic acid-treated rats', *Nutrition & Metabolism* 2010; 7: 80).

It is thought that in this way, these health-giving oils take some of the burden off the liver in terms of the toxic overload that many experience.

Whole grains

Grains, such as brown rice, are rich in B-complex vitamins, nutrients known to improve overall fat metabolism, liver function and liver decongestion. On a living foods diet, processed grains are definitely a no-no, since they are known to be associated with many degenerative conditions. However, sprouted grains, such as quinoa, amaranth, teff and buckwheat, can be a very valuable addition to the diet. Rice can be difficult to sprout, but I have successfully sprouted large-grain black rice in an automatic sprouter, so if you have one of these machines it is well worth giving it a try, since it is delicious.

Cruciferous vegetables

Eating broccoli and cauliflower will increase the amount of glucosinolate in your system, adding to enzyme production in the liver. These liver enzymes help flush out carcinogens, and other toxins, out of our body which significantly lowers our risk of cancer. Broccoli in particular is a superhero nutritionally, and if we use broccoli sprouts, the health benefits go off the charts! Broccoli contains glucoraphanin, which the body processes into the anti-cancer compound sulforaphane. This compound rids the body of *Helicobacter pylori*, a bacterium which is not only linked to gastric ulceration but also the risk of gastric cancer and even ischaemic heart disease and atrial fibrillation. Furthermore, broccoli contains indole-3-carbinol, a powerful antioxidant compound and anti-carcinogen found not only to inhibit the growth of breast, cervical and prostate cancer, but also to improve liver function.

Lemons and limes

These citrus fruits contain very high amounts of vitamin C,

which allows the body to convert toxic material into substances that are water-soluble. Drinking freshly squeezed lemon or lime juice in the morning helps to stimulate the liver, thereby acting as an aid to digestion.

Walnuts

Containing large amounts of the amino acid arginine, walnuts help the liver to detoxify ammonia. Walnuts are also high in glutathione and omega-3 fats which support normal liver cleansing actions. Make sure you soak the nuts in water for 12 hours prior to eating them, to remove the enzyme inhibitors that the nuts also contain, and chew the nuts well (until they are liquefied) before swallowing.

Cabbage

Much like broccoli and cauliflower, eating cabbage helps stimulate the activation of two crucial liver-detoxifying enzymes. Try eating fermented foods such as kimchee and sauerkraut, which are also a great source of probiotics for the bowel.

Turmeric

Turmeric is said to be the liver's favourite spice; try adding some into your next soup or dressing recipe for an instant boost. Turmeric helps to improve liver detoxification by assisting enzymes that actively flush out known dietary carcinogens.

Other foods

Other liver-cleansing foods are globe artichoke, asparagus, kale and Brussels sprouts.

Conclusion

Eating the foods listed above is a great way to keep your liver functioning properly. However, for the best results, I would recommend the liver flush protocol outlined on page 32 if you have been on a standard Western diet for a long time, provided that there are no medical contraindications.

The pancreas

The pancreas is a delicate organ that anatomically lies in a loop of the upper small intestine. It has both exocrine (digestive) and endocrine (hormonal) functions, so is another 'crossover' organ. In this section, I will be discussing the pancreas only as a digestive gland. The hormonal functions follow later, in chapter 9, notably in relation to blood sugar regulation.

The pancreas produces numerous digestive enzymes: amylase, which breaks down carbohydrates; proteases, which digest proteins; and lipase, which breaks down fats. After being manufactured in the pancreas, these enzymes transfer to the small intestine in the pancreatic juice via the pancreatic duct. Digestion of protein is initiated by pepsin in the stomach, but the bulk of the process is due to pancreatic proteases, the two major ones being trypsin and chymotrypsin.

For effective fat digestion, sufficient quantities of bile salts must also be present, so the correct digestion and assimilation of essential fats are dependent upon adequate functioning of both the liver and pancreas.

An interesting observation has been made about the pancreas: in animals fed a cooked diet, the pancreas is up to three times larger than in those given a raw food diet. This information was published in the book *Enzyme Nutrition* by Dr Edward Howell; he concluded this was because lavish enzyme secretions were needed to replace those that were missing in the cooked food, and the digestive organs were subject to enlargement (hypertrophy) as a result. It is also thought that the load put onto the pancreas by asking it to digest cooked food day in and day out is a contributing factor to pancreatic exhaustion, which some authors even suggest is a forerunner to the development of cancer (*Enzyme Therapy for Cancer and its Scientific Basis* by John Beard, 1902). Since humans are a species that traditionally cook their food, one has to wonder why it is that we do this, if it means that we are placing the burden of digestion onto our pancreatic secretions. Nobody really knows why; I guess that it is just that we have been doing it for so long, it is considered to be normal. Whether that normality goes hand in hand with optimal health is an issue that is very much open to discussion.

A recipe for good digestion: Fasting soup

I describe the benefits of fasting in chapter 11 (see page 169).This recipe, which is great for the liver and supports fasting, is one that I have adapted from the soup served at the Hippocrates Health Institute. It is a blended recipe so is very easy on the digestive system, but still contains a good source of fibre.

Quantities are approximate. Experiment with this soup to get the ratios that you prefer. Any herbs and spices can be added as extras and for increased flavour or 'warmth'.

- Spinach, celery, cucumber, lemon juice, parsley, basil, coriander leaf and avocado as a base.
- Add 250-450 ml (1-2 cups) of green juice (celery, cucumber, pea shoots & sunflower greens) depending on desired consistency (thick soup or runny soup).
- Add lots of crushed garlic for extra detox.
- Blend well in a good blender or liquidiser.
- Add cayenne and ginger for additional warmth if desired.
- Enjoy on fasting day at about 5:30pm, or for any evening meal.

Summary

- Chew your food well, or blend it if you have bad teeth
- Follow the principles of good food combining
- Get started with green juices
- Check your stomach acid levels
- Love your liver.

Chapter 3

The intestinal system

Most of the DNA in your body is not yours...

The intestinal system consists of the small and large intestine, which, following the breakdown of food via the digestive processes, are involved in the assimilation of nutrients and the elimination of waste products. The large intestine, which consists of the caecum, colon and rectum, is approximately five feet long. It is responsible for the reabsorption of many nutrients and water, and ensures normal defecation. The colon is the site where most of the absorption of water and salts takes place and vitamins are synthesised by millions of microorganisms, of which more later in this chapter.

Good functioning of the colon is fundamental to our health. In one-to-one consultations with clients, I always talk about bowel movements! Ideally, one should have a bowel movement for every meal consumed, so, if you are eating three meals a day, you should have three bowel movements a day. Apparently there are people who, in the doctor's office, inform the doctor that they are having a bowel movement once a week, and they are told that this is normal. It may be common; it is *not* normal. It is said of the UK that we are the most constipated nation in Europe. Our average transit time – that is, the time it takes for food to get from mouth to anus, is 70 hours. Seventy hours? It should be no more than 24.

It has been stated that if you have regularly eaten a standard, meat-based diet, that by the time you reach the age of 40, you have seven pounds of partially digested, rotting meat permanently lodged in your colon. This is a bad thing. Rotting meat releases very unpleasant chemicals such as skatols, which are carcinogenic. What could potentially be the outcome of this? Bowel cancer. It is on the increase in the Western world, and is more common in meat eaters than those who do not eat meat. Red and processed meats appear to be the worst offenders; indeed, in 2011, it was estimated that around 21 per cent of bowel cancers in the UK in 2010 were linked to consumption of red and processed meat (DM Parkin writing in the *British Journal of Cancer* 2011; 105(s2): s24-s26), with other studies putting the risk even higher. If you are on a diet that contains a high proportion of meat, it often follows that the fibre intake is low. Meat itself contains no dietary fibre, and fibre is vital for the correct functioning of the colon, since without it normal peristaltic movements do not occur. A high-meat, low-fibre diet is a double whammy in favour of a poorly functioning, and ultimately a diseased, colon. Sceptics might state that the traditional Inuit diet is just that (high meat, low fibre) and they have a lower incidence of chronic diseases, but this does not necessarily appear to be the case (Bjerregaard et al, 'Indigenous health in the Arctic: an overview of the circumpolar Inuit population', *Scandinavian Journal of Public Health* 2004; 32: 390-395).

The best form of fibre is found in leafy green vegetables and sprouted foods. Daily consumption of these foods will ensure that your bowel movements are sufficiently frequent and that your stool consistency is appropriate. After all, we don't want to be trying to pass bricks! I do not recommend the use of 'high fibre cereals' that are advertised as being good for bowel function. Many of these contain heavily processed grains that can cause adverse reactions as a result of their gluten content, for example. Colon health can be rapidly restored by eliminating gluten from the diet. Grain by-products, such as bran, whilst being a good source of fibre, are also known to interfere with the absorption of certain minerals, notably those which are important for bone health, so bran should not be on your menu, even if you do not have sufficiently frequent bowel movements. Psyllium husk, which comes from the seed of an Indian plant, would be far better in this instance. Psyllium is indigestible and provides soluble fibre, and is useful in the relief of constipation, additionally showing promise for reducing high cholesterol. It is available in health stores as the husk itself in its natural state, or dried and powdered.

Probiotics

It is important to consider probiotics here in regard to intestinal function. Probiotics are essentially our friendly bacteria, and we have four times as many of them as we have cells in our bodies, which is quite incredible. As I state above, most of the DNA in your body is not yours.

Here's a list of some of the recognised benefits of probiotics. They:

- Enhance the immune system response via regulating lymphocytes and antibodies
- Reduce the negative effects of taking many types of antibiotics
- Aid in preventing and treating colon inflammation
- Help to prevent eczema in youth
- Increase the ability to digest food
- Reduce lactose intolerance
- Reduce the incidence of yeast infections, vaginitis and candidiasis
- Increase the ability to assimilate the nutrients from food
- Alleviate many common digestive disorders such as constipation, diarrhoea and irritable bowel syndrome (IBS)

- Act as a remedy for bad breath (halitosis)
- Increase the ability to synthesise vitamins B and K
- Promote anti-tumour and anti-cancer activity in the body
- Improve the bio-availability of many important nutrients in the body, such as zinc, iron, phosphorus, all of the B vitamins, calcium, copper and magnesium
- Through the process of regulating intestinal transit time of faecal matter, they can dramatically reduce constipation in the elderly.

It is becoming particularly common for people to use probiotic drinks based on dairy products. I do not recommend the consumption of dairy products since I do not believe that they are a suitable food for the adult human. There is more information on this subject in my CD, *The Real Truth about Food*.

Since our probiotics represent a large percentage of our immune system, it is important to consider gut and immunity as almost one subject, rather than two separate entities. If your immune function is poor, a course of probiotics would be an excellent idea.

What goes on in the colon?

The colon is an important part of the human body, and at present, it appears to be the focus of intense interest. It is of the utmost importance to know more about this previously neglected part of the digestive tract. Your health depends on it.

It is the site where most of the absorption of water and salts takes place and vitamins are synthesised by millions of microorganisms.

Some food components, such as dietary fibre and oligosaccharides, which escape digestion in the upper parts of the digestive tract, are exposed to bacterial digestion in the colon. The colonic microflora, as these 'good' microorganisms are called, not only digest otherwise indigestible food components, but also manufacture a variety of significant vitamins which can be utilised by the human body.

Vitamin synthesis

The microflora of the colon synthesise the following vitamins:

- Vitamin K – essential for blood clotting and bone health
- Vitamin B12 – prevents pernicious or megaloblastic anaemia
- Thiamine (B1) and riboflavin (B2) – play an important role in most metabolic processes (energy release), keep the nervous system functioning optimally and help to lower homocysteine levels, which are implicated in heart disease (see chapter 4, page xxx).

After synthesis, these vitamins (apart from vitamin B12, which can only be absorbed in the ileum, when combined with intrinsic factor) are absorbed through the wall of the colon for use in the body. Those with poor colonic health might be compromising their absorption of vitamins B1, B2 and K.

Production of short-chain fatty acids

The microflora of the colon also ferment otherwise indigestible food components to produce short-chain fatty acids (SCFAs). The SCFAs provide fuel for the colonocytes (cells of the colon) and help with the absorption of water and salts.

Boosting immunity

The colon and its microflora also help to boost immunity. Recent research has shown that a healthy population of various microorganisms, such as *Lactobacilli*, and *Bifidobacteria*, can contribute to general health and increase our resistance to various infections (*Candida, Salmonella, Escherichia coli*).

Cholesterol lowering

Research has demonstrated that diets rich in soluble fibre (pectins from fruit, and hemicellulose from fruit, oats, legumes and psyllium) are capable of lowering raised blood cholesterol levels. Two theories have been suggested to explain this finding: either the soluble fibre in the colon binds bile acids, which are produced by the gall bladder, so that additional cholesterol has to be used up to produce more bile acids, or the microflora in the colon ferment the soluble fibre to SCFAs, which inhibit cholesterol production in the body.

What does a healthy colon require?

A healthy colon requires the following nutrients:
- Plenty of **soluble dietary fibre** – fruit, oats, and sprouted legumes to bind bile acids and lower blood cholesterol levels
- Plenty of **insoluble dietary fibre** (plant fibre) to promote regularity
- **Oligosaccharides** – Jerusalem artichokes, asparagus, onions, garlic and mushrooms, plus nutraceuticals (e.g. foods containing inulin and other oligosaccharides), which promote the viability of colonic microflora
- **Microflora supplements** (probiotics), which contain *Lactobacilli* or *Bifidobacteria*, to increase the number of 'good' bacteria in the colon
- Water to help dietary fibre swell up and promote peristalsis to regulate bowel movements.

Factors that disturb the health of the colon

Colon health is relatively easily disturbed by any of the following factors:

- Diets with a low fibre content consisting of highly processed starches, protein and fat
- Antibiotics, which destroy the microflora
- Excessive stress
- Infections causing diarrhoea
- Use of harsh chemical and herbal laxatives
- High meat consumption.

These factors, alone or in combination, can either destroy the microflora, thus allowing harmful bacteria and yeasts (*Candida*) to take over and proliferate, or damage the normal peristalsis of the colon.

As an aid to restoration of colonic health, the Hippocrates Health Institute (see page xxx) advises 'enemas and implants', and all guests at the Institute are encouraged to perform these twice daily. A high warm-water enema is taken, then eliminated. Following this, a wheatgrass juice implant is inserted into the colon and held, if possible, until full absorption has taken place. The wheatgrass juice feeds the natural probiotics of the bowel and helps to restore the integrity of an inflamed colonic wall. You can find a step-by-step guide to how to do it in my e-book *Successful Fasting for Health and Vitality*. If you have any known colonic health issues, always check with your medical practitioner first that this procedure is suitable for you.

For a colon that is very badly diseased, a course of 'colonics' is also advisable. Colonic hydrotherapy differs from an enema in that larger volumes of water are used under pressure, and more of the colon is flushed. The practice is very beneficial for someone whose diet has consisted of a large amount of meat, in which there may be accumulated pockets of undesirable waste material. If you have never experienced a colonic before, don't panic; it is not a dirty or unpleasant experience. Seek out a sympathetic practitioner or go on personal recommendation.

If you have ulcerative colitis or Crohn's Disease, take professional advice first. An implant which has been specifically found to help with such inflammatory disorders includes aloe vera juice and fenugreek sprout juice, but check with your medical professional first to ensure that this is appropriate for you.

An alternative option for those who feel unable to do enemas, implants or colonics would be a product called Internal Cleanser. This is made by the Hippocrates Health Institute and can be obtained via the Institute itself, or again via Antidote in the UK (see page 189 for resources).

A recipe for intestinal health: Chia seed porridge

Despite its potentially unappetising appearance, chia porridge is absolutely full of beneficial nutrients and I firmly believe that the tiny chia seed should be on the regular menu of all serious health seekers. Ensure that you allow time, before eating this porridge, for the chia seeds to swell up as they take on the liquid. They expand to up to 10 times their original size, and it's better that this occurs in the breakfast bowl rather than in your stomach.

Ingredients
250 ml (1 cup) pure water
1 tablespoonful raw almond butter (or raw rainforest butter)
4 dates, stone removed (or a pinch of stevia powder if you're sugar-free)
½ teaspoon vanilla powder
Your choice of superfood powder (optional)
2 tablespoons chia seeds

- Place the water, dates/stevia and raw nut butter in a blender.
- Blend on a medium setting until well combined.
- If using dates, you might need a high setting to ensure the resulting nut milk is smooth. Alternatively soak the dates overnight in water beforehand.
- If you're using a superfood or food supplement powder, add this at the end and blend for 5-10 seconds only on a very low speed.
- This gives you your nut milk.
- Put the chia seeds in a breakfast bowl and pour on your nut milk, stirring to prevent the seeds from floating.
- Leave the seeds to soak in the nut milk for about 15 minutes, stirring occasionally, until they swell up and you are left with a porridge consistency.
- Enjoy after a long run or heavy gym session.

Summary

- Probiotics are your new best friend
- You should have one bowel movement for every meal you eat
- The colon often needs to be cleansed to become fully healthy
- Meat, dairy products and processed grains aggravate the colon.

Chapter 4

The circulatory system

One pump, more than 60,000 miles of pipework.

The circulatory system exists simply to move that wondrous fluid, blood, around our bodies. Many state that blood truly is the 'fluid of life', and it would be hard to disagree. In the case of our red blood cells, I certainly believe that Mother Nature, or evolution, had a day of genius when they were developed. They do not contain a nucleus, which means that more haemoglobin, the oxygen-carrying molecule in the blood, can be packed in. Their structure, in biology known as a 'bi-concave disc', enables the cells to be slightly deformed as they pass through the tiniest vessels, and also present a greater surface area for exchange than a totally flat cell would have. What a brilliant design.

The circulatory system consists of a pump (the four-chambered heart) and the pipes – arteries, which carry oxygenated blood to all the tissues via the smaller arterioles and capillaries, and veins, which return the blood to the heart from the tissues. Arteries have elastic, muscular walls to enable them to withstand the pressure generated by each heartbeat. Veins have very little elastic tissue in their walls, and contain valves to ensure that the blood in them flows only in one direction.

With our circulatory system, we want to think about not only the cells themselves that carry the oxygen, but also the fluid part of the blood, and the many miles of pipework along which this life-sustaining fluid passes. We want to 'build the blood' for greater health, but what exactly does that mean, and how do we do it?

Meet your blood

Blood is made up of three distinct parts:
- Red and white blood cells
- Plasma
- Platelets.

Red blood cells

The red blood cells, as stated, are responsible for the carriage of oxygen. The white blood cells are involved in immunity. The plasma is the fluid component of the blood, and allows the cells to flow freely. Platelets are responsible for blood clotting. The cells make up approximately 45 per cent of blood volume.

Anything that affects the formation of cells in general, either positively or negatively, will in turn affect the blood. Foods rich in chlorophyll, the green component of plants, are best for blood-building: it has been demonstrated in numerous human and animal trials that fresh wheatgrass juice can reverse anaemia (low red blood cell count). It is interesting to look at the chemical structure of chlorophyll and compare it to that of haemoglobin in Figure 3 – you will see that the molecules are very similar.

There are many reasons why the cereal grasses, such as wheatgrass, and other dark green plants can be considered 'blood-building' foods. Nutrients essential to the maintenance of healthy blood include iron, copper, calcium, vitamins A, C, B12, K, folic acid and pyridoxine; all of these nutrients are abundant in the green foods and wheatgrass juice. The vitamins and minerals in wheatgrass are essential to the synthesis and function of the components of healthy blood. However, perhaps the most inter-esting connection between green foods and blood remains the

Haeme
(Oxygen-carrying portion
of haemoglobin)

Chlorophyll

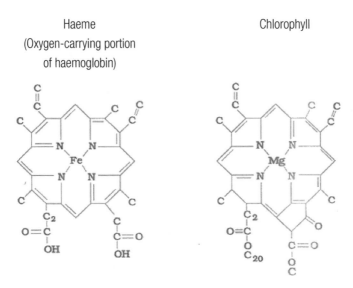

Figure 3: Comparison of haeme and chlorophyll molecules. Note that haeme has an iron (Fe) ion in the middle and chlorophyll has a magnesium (Mg) ion in a very similar structure

similarity in the structures of the two coloured pigments, haeme and chlorophyll. The biological relationship between these two molecules, though studied for over 60 years, is still not completely clear. It does appear, however, that small amounts of the digestive products of chlorophyll may stimulate the synthesis of either haeme or globin or both in animals, including humans. The metabolic pathway is probably more complicated than just swopping a magnesium ion for an iron ion to turn chlorophyll into haemoglobin, but the 'life blood' of plants is definitely closely related to, and beneficial for, the life blood of humans.

White blood cells are considerably less numerous than the red blood cells in the circulation. The white blood cells are fundamentally involved with the functioning of the immune system, which is discussed in chapter 6.

Platelets

Platelets are involved in the processes of blood clotting and wound healing. Whilst blood clotting is an essential bodily mechanism, it can occur inappropriately, with potentially disastrous consequences, depending upon where in the body the blood clot occurs. Since platelet agglutination (sticking-together of platelets) is a major risk factor for both heart attack and stroke, modern medicine is keen to provide us with drugs that reduce this risk, with aspirin being one. However, there are drug-free alternatives which may be just as effective, and without the side-effects, such as garlic (Gadkari JV, Joshi VD, 'Effect of raw garlic on serum cholesterol level, clotting time and fibrinolytic activity in normal subjects', *Journal of Postgraduate Medicine* 1991; 37(23): 128-131), but it seems that the garlic must be eaten raw to achieve these benefits (Bordia et al, 'An evaluation of garlic and onion as antithrombotic agents', *Prostaglandins Leukotrienes and Essent Fatty Acids* 1996; 54(3): 183-186). Ultimately, to ensure that our platelets behave as they should, it is important to eat a diet which has already been proven to reduce the risk of heart attacks – that is, one based on plants, with a high intake of fresh vegetables and naturally occurring antioxidants (Iqbal R, Anand S, Ounpuu S et al, 'Dietary patterns and the risk of acute myocardial infarction in 52 countries: results of the INTERHEART study', *Circulation* 2008; 118(19): 1913-1914).

Plasma and general circulation

Dehydration will reduce the total volume of blood plasma, and will cause the cell volume to rise relative to the plasma volume. If the packed cell volume rises to over 50 per cent of the total blood volume, the oxygen-carrying capacity of the red blood cells can be reduced as they may start to stack upon one another. Thicker blood also means that the flow will be adversely affected, so it is important to pay attention to hydration status, as discussed in chapter 8 (see page 103).

Several factors affect the circulation, including the heart rate, fitness level, stroke volume (amount of blood the heart ejects after each beat), exercise levels, blood thickness, elasticity of arterial walls, any build-up of cholesterol plaque from consuming animal products, dehydration... a long list.

In addition to the information given in chapter 2 regarding the lemon water with cayenne (see page 21), there are many ways in which the circulation can be improved.

My recommendations for improved circulation always start with increasing the exercise levels, which, in addition to having benefits for the circulatory system, positively affects brain chemistry, making us feel happier. Exercise is also essential for gaining muscle strength; it speeds the metabolism and prevents us from feeling cold. Finally, it is of huge benefit for the structural integrity of the bones (osteoporosis prevention). Ideally we all need to aim for 30 minutes five times a week. Exercise should be at a level which will make you breathe heavily but still be able to hold a conversation, but not be able to sing. Walking, swimming and using a mini trampoline are all great ways to exercise. All of these are excellent for cardiovascular health, and low impact, thereby not causing excess stress on the joints. The most important thing is finding something you enjoy doing. Even vigorous housecleaning and gardening have benefits. People often ask me what the best form of exercise is. My reply is always the same – the one that you will do. Make sure you build up slowly at first with any exercise if you're not used to it.

More advanced exercise strategies that I recommend for the fitness enthusiast or athlete include sprint training, using either a treadmill, cross trainer, rowing machine or bike. This can be as hard as you want to make it, and is a fantastic way of building strength, stamina and speed whilst reducing the actual amount of time that you need to spend exercising. We are all busy these days, but a sprint workout can be completed in just 20 minutes, and we've all got time to do that, haven't we?

I mention to my clients that 75 per cent of the benefits of an excellent diet are lost if they don't exercise. That gives you an indication of just how important it is to keep moving.

If we have poor circulation, there is less oxygen delivered to all our body tissues. This is of vital importance since lack of oxygen to the brain will cause foggy thinking, lack of blood delivered to the intestines will inhibit our capacity to absorb nutrients, lack of blood to the muscles will affect our ability to exercise, and the reduced tissue oxygenation that occurs with, for example, smoking and poor circulation increases cancer risk, because cancer cells thrive in anaerobic conditions. As long ago as 1936, Nobel Laureate Otto Warburg published a scientific paper called *The Ultimate Cause of Cancer*, which indicated that if cells were deprived of 60 per cent of their oxygen for 36 hours, they automatically became cancerous. Never underestimate the importance of cellular oxygenation for health.

As we have seen, green drinks and juices are perfect for increasing tissue oxygenation, as they contain a large amount of chlorophyll. They also ensure that you will remain well hydrated. As described in chapter 1, I always recommend a large green juice every day, preferably for breakfast, for long-term use. Why not try it (see page 19)? I do hope that this will become part of your routine from now on – it really is one of the best ways to kick-start a healthy lifestyle.

Another recommendation for cardiovascular health that I make is Juice Plus Vineyard capsules. Studies have shown that they improve the elasticity and blood-carrying capacity of the arteries after a high-fat meal, and additionally the berries and grapes present in the capsules contain the vast array of anti-oxidants which have proven benefits for cardiovascular health, even in smokers. This is like having the benefits of red grape skins in wine, without the alcohol, sulphites, sugar and all the other damaging factors present in wine. (For those not ready to leave red wine behind, Chilean Merlot wine has been shown to contain higher levels of certain antioxidants than those grown in other countries (Faustino et al, 'Comparative analysis of the phenolic content of selected Chilean, Canadian and American Merlot red wines', *Molecular Cell Biochemistry*. 2003; 249(1-2): 11-9). However, remember that alcohol in any quantity destroys brain cells and compromises liver function. Using Juice Plus as a food supplement has been demonstrated to have many other benefits for health in addition to its positive results for the circulation. Studies have shown that it improves the immune system, decreases DNA damage, increases VO2Max (a measurement of the ability to transport and use oxygen during exercise) in athletes, improves oral health, reduces biomarkers of ageing and prevents pre-eclampsia (high blood pressure) in pregnant women, to name a few. See appendix 2 for a comprehensive list of the published studies.

We know a lot about the beneficial effects of plant consumption on the circulatory system (further outlined below), but we also need to consider what is harmful to our cardiovascular function. Good reasons to totally avoid both smoking and eating animal products include their adverse effects on the circulation due to increasing cholesterol plaque and the secondary effect of deposition of animal protein in the vascular basement membrane, which causes a reduction in the elasticity of the vessels and their subsequent narrowing. For more information on this subject, listen to my CD *The Real Truth About Food*.

Foods that may help your circulation

Let's review some foods that are considered to be beneficial for the circulation:

Dark chocolate: It is often stated in the 'health literature' that chocolate is good for the circulation, and there are many in the raw food world who continue to insist that raw chocolate is a superfood. Whilst natural, unprocessed cacao contains important flavonols that improve blood circulation and ward off blood clots associated with stroke and heart attacks, these elements can also be found in other foods, such as blueberries (see below). Whilst raw cacao is also a good source of magnesium, it is often not eaten alone. Many raw chocolate confections contain a lot of fat and added sugar, often in the form of agave syrup, which is as bad for the body as high-fructose corn syrup. Be aware also that cacao, whether raw or cooked, contains caffeine, theophylline and theobromine, which are all stimulants and can adversely affect the adrenal glands. If you fancy a bit of raw dark chocolate, don't let me stop you, but see it as the recreational treat that it is, and not a superfood that you need on a daily basis.

Blueberries and **grapes** contain heart-healthy flavonoids and resveratrol that protect us from free radicals that damage and attack healthy cells. They also improve the metabolism. Resveratrol has also been shown to stimulate sirtuins, recently discovered genes that are responsible for longevity – what a bonus.

Oranges: Citrus fruit in general are considered to be high in vitamin C which has artery-strengthening properties and also prevents plaque build-up. This is true, but oranges are not 'top of the pops' for vitamin C content – that honour goes to the camu camu berry, an Amazonian fruit which is sometimes incorporated into whole-food supplements. Don't let that put you off citrus fruit though – they are easy to get hold of, whereas camu-camu is not, and they still have many health benefits.

Avocados: Rich in heart-healthy fats, they support the cardiovascular system. One cup of avocado has 23 per cent of the recommended daily value of folate. Studies show that people who eat diets rich in folate have a much lower incidence of heart disease than those who don't. The vitamin E, monounsaturated fats, and glutathione in avocado are also great for your heart.

Cayenne pepper: This powerful spice is a great way to increase blood circulation and metabolic rate, whilst also helping to strengthen arteries and blood vessels, preventing poor circulation in the extremities. Cayenne pepper is the most effective taken raw in salads or juiced; adjust the heat level according to your preference.

Ginger: This warming root stimulates the blood flow to all organs; it also boosts a sluggish immune system and clears congestion.

Garlic is fantastic for increasing blood circulation in the extremities, and will also clear up clogged arteries if eaten raw daily. Garlic also has many benefits for the immune system and is antiviral and antifungal. It thins the blood and has been shown to lower cholesterol as effectively as cholesterol-reducing medications, with none of the adverse side effects. Raw garlic can be added to your daily green juice and can be crushed onto salads. Use 1-2 cloves per meal for best effects.

Gingko biloba is a herb used by Chinese health practitioners to increase blood circulation. It improves poor circulation in the hands and feet, is used to treat varicose veins and increases blood flow to the brain.

Pumpkin seeds: These tasty seeds contain high levels of vitamin E, proven to keep blood flowing freely and preventing blood clots.

Omega-3: It is stated by many that salmon and other oily types of fish, which are very high in omega-3 fatty acids, should be eaten to improve blood circulation, and we have probably all seen adverts telling us that we should take fish-oil capsules for a healthy heart. However, it is known that due to high levels of environmental pollution, large fish that are high in the food chain contain many toxic elements, including mercury and organophosphates. Farmed fish are contaminated with the antibiotics and other chemicals which are added to the water they swim in, making them unsuitable for consumption by the health seeker.

For more information on the concerns about fish eating, I suggest reading *Killer Fish*, by Brian Clement.

A good plant source of omega-3 oils is flax oil, but this, still, does not contain the DHA (docosahexaenoic acid) and EPA (eicosapentaenoic acid) that fish oil contains. Fish obtain these fats from the algae they eat, so by 'cutting out the middle fish', we can obtain these beneficial oils from blue-green algae, such as E3 Live (see resources section).

In addition to the foods above, if you experience poor circulation, a great solution can be contrast showers when you switch water temperatures from warm to cold and vice versa. Conversely, caffeine, alcohol and smoking can dramatically constrict the blood flow to the heart and organs and should be avoided by everyone.

Arterial cleansing

Finally, before we leave the subject of the circulatory system, let us look at the potential effectiveness of an arterial cleansing programme. It has always amused me to think that there are many heart surgeons performing bypass operations and removing just a few centimetres of clogged-up coronary artery, when it is in fact the whole 60,000 miles or so of the circulatory system that will be clogged up with arterial plaque. Reduced arterial flow affects all the pipes equally. Particularly significant for men in this regard is erectile dysfunction; an arterial cleansing programme will rapidly normalise this distressing condition.

The main reason that bypass operations are performed is that blockage of a coronary artery can lead to sudden death, whereas in other parts of the body the effects are not acutely life-threatening but are seen as longer-term chronic degeneration.

What does an arterial cleansing programme involve? Firstly, a low-protein vegan diet needs to be adopted. When animal protein is eaten, particularly in larger quantities, the body has no easy way of processing it all, so it uses the vascular basement membrane as a kind of 'protein dump'. Over time, the result is a gradual stiffening of this membrane and narrowing of the associated artery. A low-protein diet that excludes all animal protein will immediately prevent further protein deposition in the vascular basement membrane. Additionally, I recommend the use of proteolytic enzymes. This special type of enzyme breaks down stored proteins and scarring of the arterial walls and over time allows for renewed elasticity of the vessels.

By adopting a standard vegan diet that includes only 1 per cent protein, it has been demonstrated that the blood vessels can be cleared out in four months. If we adopt a living-foods vegan diet, and use whole-food supplementation and proteolytic enzymes, the problem can be reversed much faster than this. The fastest recovery I ever saw in a client took just three weeks; it involved the Hippocrates dietary regime, supplemented with colon cleansing, lots of extra garlic and the use of Vitalzym and the full range of Juice Plus capsules (see page 182). I call this 'bypassing the bypass' – and the gentleman concerned has not only completely avoided the need for heart surgery, but has also reversed other degenerative changes noted on his blood profile, lost over 40 pounds (18 kilos) in weight and has taken up running, all to the amazement of his doctors. Yes, the regime could be considered to be radical, but so is cutting open the chest and transplanting blood vessels. And remember that heart and bypass surgery, brilliant as it is, does not actually address the original reason that the bypass was needed; unless the patient changes his or her diet, the vessels will just block up again. When you are staring imminent death in the face, you often have to be pretty radical with your choices. For more transformational stories of healing and disease reversal, I recommend reading *LifeForce*, by Dr Brian Clement.

Filtering the blood

This the job of the spleen. It filters the blood to take out all the old worn-out red blood cells and then destroys them. They are replaced by new red blood cells that are made in the bone marrow. The spleen also filters out bacteria, viruses and other foreign particles found in the blood. White blood cells in the spleen attack bacteria and viruses as they pass through.

The lymphatic system

No discussion on circulation would be complete without mentioning the lymphatic system. At the level of our capillaries, some of the blood plasma leaks out into the tissues. This leakage is an important part of our cellular processes since it carries nutrients into the cells and in turn allows cellular wastes to be transported back to the blood stream. The leaked fluid drains back into the lymphatic vessels, is filtered by the lymphatic glands, and then empties back into the venous circulation via the thoracic duct, in the upper part of the chest.

Surprisingly, at any one time, there is four times as much lymphatic fluid in circulation in your body than there is blood. The lymphatic system is part of the circulation and consists of lymph vessels plus lymphatic glands, which are at strategic places anatomically. The lymphatic glands also play a big part in immunity, so again we can see that we cannot just consider each body system in its own right; they are all intricately connected with each other.

The flow of lymphatic fluid is largely governed by muscular movements during exercise, and helps to explain why people who are largely sedentary may develop swollen ankles if sitting for too long.

Two excellent ways to stimulate the flow of the lymph are rebounding on a mini trampoline, and dry skin brushing, using movements towards the heart. There is also a massage technique known as lymphatic drainage massage which is excellent for stimulating the flow of lymph fluid back towards the heart. Most qualified massage therapists will be able to perform this technique for you.

The lymphatic system has a number of functions:

Filtering lymph: The lymph nodes filter the lymph fluid as it passes through. White blood cells attack any bacteria or viruses they find in the lymph as it flows through the lymph nodes.

Fighting infection: The lymphatic system helps to fight infection in many ways, including by producing lymphocytes, a type of white blood cell that in turn produces antibodies, and via macrophages, another type of white blood cell that is present in the lymph glands and ingests and kills foreign invaders.

A recipe for your circulation: Fiery sweet potatoes

This recipe is an all-time favourite of mine. Spicy, warming and filling, 'FSPs', as I call them, are a great accompaniment to a kale salad on a cold day.

Ingredients
1-2 tablespoons olive oil
2 teaspoons Tamari or Nama Shoyu (raw soy sauce)
1 tablespoon minced garlic
1 tablespoon minced ginger root
½ teaspoon dried red chilli, or half a fresh red chilli
½ teaspoon cayenne pepper
1-2 tablespoons pure water
2 large (3 cups) grated sweet potatoes

- Blend the oil, tamari, garlic, ginger and cayenne until it's a smooth mixture. Add additional water if needed to achieve the desired consistency.
- Place sweet potatoes in a bowl and pour dressing over, stirring in before serving.
- This is great as an accompaniment to salad, or on its own as a filling snack or meal in its own right.

Summary

- Exercise is essential for good circulation
- Garlic, ginger and cayenne improve the blood flow
- Meat and dairy products impair blood flow via deposition of atherosclerotic plaque
- Atherosclerosis can be reversed via a vascular cleansing protocol
- Chlorophyll-rich foods (greens) help to build the blood
- The lymphatics are involved in both circulatory and immune systems.

Chapter 5

The nervous system

Your brain, and 45 miles of nerves.

The nervous system is a huge area to consider, and yet again we find that it influences the other body systems, notably the immune system. Indeed, it really does appear that 'thoughts are things'.

The nervous system can be broadly divided into the central nervous system, which comprises the brain and spinal cord, and the peripheral nervous system, consisting of nerves which connect the central nervous system to every other part of the body. The peripheral nervous system includes the autonomic nervous system (divisible further into the sympathetic and para-sympathetic systems), and is considered largely to be outside voluntary control, although the boundaries may be blurred somewhat as we discover what is possible through advanced meditation practice, for example. I go into a lot of detail about feeding the brain in my CD/MP3 of the same title, available on my website, so I have given just a basic summary below.

I have always been fascinated by human potential, par-ticularly any aspect which relates to the brain. I have met people who have reached beyond the age of 100 who were still able to enjoy wit and conversation with those 80 years their junior, and marvelled how they managed to keep their minds sharp and agile, whilst others seemed to experience just the opposite – a premature fading of their mental faculties. I certainly intend to be in the former category when I hold my 100th birthday party on the beach in Hawaii in January 2063, and ensure that I can go surfing with everyone else. Whilst some may say that I am being overoptimistic with my birthday plans, I don't see why it shouldn't be possible. After all, wasn't it Paul Bragg who famously died in a surfing accident aged 109, with a brain that was as active as that of most people in their 20s? If you want to do the same, let's consider the 10 things you absolutely must do if you want a fit and agile brain to go with a fit and agile body.

1. Oxygenate

Oxygen is the most important brain nutrient by far. We can last weeks without food, days without water, but only minutes without air. Ensure that you oxygenate your body and brain by deep breathing in clean environments, avoiding air pollution wherever possible, cleaning up your indoor air with 'green' cleaning products and houseplants (see chapter 11, page 171), and exercising regularly. Get into nature whenever you can, and focus on your breathing. Grow wheatgrass in your house. However you do it, get some good clean air into your lungs.

2. Eat your greens

As I describe in chapter 4, green foods build the blood. The reason is chlorophyll, the molecule that gives plants their lovely bright green colour and is our best friend in regard to oxygenation. The foods highest in chlorophyll are the foods that give us the greatest tissue oxygenation potential – including wheatgrass juice, blue green algae and sunflower greens. Use them every day to help to oxygenate your body. Leafy green salads also contain chlorophyll, but not as much as wheatgrass and the algae.

3. Hydrate!

Altogether 80 per cent of the brain is water. If we are dehydrated, the brain won't function properly. Ensure you are well hydrated by drinking half a fluid ounce of water for every pound of your bodyweight every day. Drink only pure water (not chlorinated or out of a plastic bottle; see chapter 8, page 104 for why we should avoid plastic water bottles) and low glycaemic vegetable juices. 'Glycaemic', here, relates to the rate at which sugar is absorbed. Foods with a low glycaemic index (GI) do not cause 'spikes' in blood sugar levels, and therefore avoid insulin surges (see page 70). Cucumber juice is a fantastic way of hydrating yourself, as is coconut water (the juice inside fresh coconuts). Avoid coffee and standard tea. Herb teas are a good substitute for regular tea and coffee. Ignore claims that 'coffee is good for you' with the contempt that they deserve. As for 'sports drinks', please see my explanation of their failings in chapter 9.

4. Preserve your enzymes

As I explain in chapter 4, enzymes are the chemicals all living organisms produce to enable chemical processes to take place within the body. Several studies, notably those collated in the books *Enzyme Nutrition: The Food Enzyme Concept* by Dr Edward Howell, and *Enzymes: The Fountain of Life* by K Miehlke, RM Williams and DA Lopez, have indicated that by eating food in its raw state, with the enzymes intact, atherosclerotic plaque can be cleared from the arteries. This, in turn, allows better blood flow to all parts of the body, thereby giving better tissue oxygenation. The standard Western diet, high in meat, dairy products and processed grains, reduces blood flow by narrowing the arteries over time.

5. Eat brightly coloured plants in their raw state

Brightly coloured fruit and vegetables contain a huge spectrum of antioxidants and phytonutrients, many of which probably don't even have names yet. It has been estimated that there are perhaps 25,000 different antioxidants in the plants that we eat, so there's no way that we could ever expect a regular 'antioxidant supplement' to contain all of the elements that we need for brain health, or indeed the health of any other body part. Studies in both dogs and humans have indicated that oxidative stress is one of the main factors involved in brain ageing. This can successfully be reversed using whole food antioxidant supplementation and basing the diet on whole, ripe, raw vegetables and fruit, rather than meat and dairy, which contain no beneficial antioxidants.

6. Avoid hypoglycaemia (low blood sugar)

Low blood sugar causes the brain to malfunction. A cautious estimate is that over 60 per cent of people in the Western world have blood sugar regulation difficulties. Pancreatic exhaustion is becoming more and more common, and increasingly in young people. It is not just age-related. Base your diet on good-quality plant protein and low-glycaemic vegetables and fruit, and all but the most stubborn forms of sugar regulation will disappear. I cover this in more detail later in this chapter.

7. Have something to do

Get a hobby! Exercise your brain by getting active and involved in your community. Meet people in different age groups from yourself. Learn a new language (you do have time, and it's fun), play games such as chess that stimulate the mind. A wise man once told me that, 'You need something to do, something to look forward to and someone to love.' How true.

8. Exercise

As I say in every chapter, 75 per cent of the benefit of a good diet is wasted without exercise. For maximum brain-boosting, lift weights. Studies show that weight training stimulates the parts of the brain that are usually first affected by Alzheimer's.

Perform weight-training exercises and you'll have a more functional brain and you'll look sexier. What could be better?

9. Avoid the 'bad stuff'

Many factors are known for their brain-diminishing properties. Here are 13 of them that you absolutely must avoid if you want your brain to work properly, so that we can have a stimulating conversation when you come to my 100th birthday party.

Psychotropic drugs	Environmental pollutants
Coffee	Lack of good quality sleep
Alcohol	Refined sugar
Standard Western diets	Aluminium
Mercury	Artificial sweeteners (e.g.
Smoking	aspartame)
Stress	Mobile phones.

There's a good reason for listing all of these. You'll find more information on each in my CD/MP3 *Feeding the Brain*.

10. Cultivate a positive attitude

Happiness can appear to be that most elusive of emotions, but this is probably the most important of all factors and has a massive impact not only on our brain function, but on our overall health levels and experience of life. Seek out positive people and enjoy their company. Avoid the naysayers. There's more than enough gloom and doom in the media, so switch off the TV and go outside and play, whatever your age. Laugh, have fun, share and be grateful for what you have.

The nervous system is incredibly complex, and can be very much affected by food and lifestyle factors. The two main areas I like to think about in this regard are blood sugar regulation (as already touched on with 'hypoglycaemia') and alkalising. Each of these has the ability to improve brain function, which is important for anyone who suffers mood swings, irritation, tiredness depression or any one of a host of other 21st-century ailments.

One of the best ways of incorporating the benefits of both alkalising and blood sugar regulation is the daily green juice, taken each morning. The sprouted sunflower greens and pea shoots contain a complete spectrum of proteins (see chapter 1, page 3), and the sunflower greens have a massive Kirlian field (see page 3), essential for healing and restoration of energy. The cucumber is very hydrating and the celery provides organic minerals, which feed the adrenal glands. (The adrenals are often exhausted in stressed individuals.) Good protein balance is essential for stabilisation of blood sugar. After several weeks on a green juice regime, people really start to notice a difference in their energy levels and their nervous system begins to function better.

Better blood sugar regulation can be rapidly achieved by incorporating more living food into the diet, since salads, vegetables and sprouted foods are all low on the GI scale. Conversely, a diet high in processed grains, bread, cakes, biscuits, confectionery and even 'raw' cakes, sweet treats and dried fruit, will reduce the ability to smooth out insulin surges, thereby allowing higher 'peaks' and lower 'troughs' in blood glucose levels. Remember that what you drink is important too. Devoid of fibre, fruit juices are not actually considered to be a healthy choice; you're better off eating the whole fruit, or having a green juice instead. Ideally, to avoid hyper- and hypoglycaemia, fresh fruit juices should be diluted one in 10 with water. Drinks with added sugar are even worse, and should be avoided by everyone. Canned, carbonated drinks are the worst of all, and have no place on a health-seeker's menu.

To allow for better and more restful sleep, which rejuvenates the nervous system, I recommend that people do not eat too close to bedtime. Many have a challenge with this, since we are all creatures of habit and often we are used to eating at a certain time of day. Ideally one should eat the evening meal three hours before bed, which would mean eating no later than 7 pm if you go to bed at 10 pm. For bed-time relaxation, I have found valerian tea to be beneficial for my clients. It is safe and non habit-forming.

Do you meditate? Meditation is a fantastic tool for health, and has been shown to have widespread benefits when performed on a regular basis. It has also been shown by neuroscientists to stimulate areas of the brain that are responsible for the production of feelings of happiness. Some of the happiest people I know are committed meditators. Meditation is also really good for those whose nervous systems are out of whack, and is well known to be a drug-free way of lowering blood pressure whilst also increasing tissue oxygenation, if combined with proper breathing techniques. If there is a meditation group close to where you live, join in. It's also worth contacting your local adult education centre to find out about group practice. At first, you might find it a bit tricky; after all, it is an acquired skill and can only be perfected, like anything else, with regular practice. I, for one, am hopeless at sitting still cross legged on the floor and trying to clear my brain. However, even I can do it – I just cheat and use a guided visualisation. This has the same effect but is easier to get to grips with. I recommend that if you are getting a guided visualisation CD, you choose someone with a nice voice, otherwise you'll end up more irritated than relaxed. I personally like Chrissy White's CD for this (see the resources section at the end of this book).

Do persevere with your practice. Recent studies have shown that regular meditation improves immune responses and lessens the likelihood of coming down with winter illnesses, for example. Think of meditation as one of the 'keys' that will unlock the door to better mental agility and greater feelings of well-being, but don't forget that there are others. In this category I include long-distance running (some of the best mind-calming effects I have had have been whilst running) and t'ai chi, so if you don't, for whatever reason, find that meditation works for you after giving it a good try, consider other keys which will allow you to open the same door. As stated in the book *Destructive Emotions*, a summary of collaborations between neuroscientists and the Dalai Lama, that key may be made of gold, silver or iron, but the door will be opened nonetheless.

Brain food

There are some nutrients that are worthy of separate mention in relation to the central nervous system. The living foods diet will be high in all of these nutrients, but the following, in my opinion, are worth additional overview.

Thiamine-containing foods

Your brain relies on thiamine (vitamin B1) to produce neuro-transmitters, which are needed to send messages throughout your nervous system. Without adequate thiamine, people can experience brain-related symptoms such as loss of memory and even brain damage. Conventional eaters are usually told to eat cereals and grains that are minimally processed, such as whole-wheat breads or brown rice, and to eat fortified cereals. However, always looking for ways in which to upgrade, I prefer the sources found in a living foods regime, in which the sprouted small grains such as quinoa, amaranth and teff serve your needs. Soaked nuts (see page 165) and sprouted legumes (see page 16) are also good dietary sources.

Potassium-containing foods

Your brain relies on potassium to generate the chemical reactions that create energy and allow your brain cells to communicate. If you don't get enough potassium in your daily diet, you can experience symptoms such as mental confusion and even an irregular heartbeat. Fruits and vegetables tend to be highest in potassium; we all think of bananas as being high in potassium, but all the dark-green foods are great sources.

Zinc-containing foods

Your body requires zinc each day to improve your memory and keep you thinking clearly, and a good source is soaked pumpkin seeds, and pumpkin seed butter. Eating a handful of these seeds, ideally soaked before eating them, can give you all the zinc you need to boost your brain power. Sprouted lentils and chick peas (garbanzo beans) are also good sources of zinc. See how easy it is?

High-calcium foods

While you may think of calcium as a mineral that strengthens your bones and teeth, your brain requires calcium to transmit nerve signals. On the living foods diet we are never thinking about dairy products as a source of calcium (see chapter 10 about the structural system), so remember that dark-green leafy foods such as kale will give you plenty of calcium, as will raw tahini (see the resources section, page 197).

Magnesium-containing foods

Magnesium, a crucial dietary mineral, helps maintain proper cardiovascular system function, affects energy metabolism and plays a part in bone health. Magnesium also helps maintain the health of the nervous system. In their book, *Psychiatric Side Effects of Prescription and Over-the-Counter Medications: Recognition and Management*, doctors Thomas Markham Brown and Alan Stoudemire report that magnesium has an inhibitory effect on certain neurotransmitters, the brain chemicals responsible for signal transmission between nerve cells. Specifically, magnesium helps with the manufacture of dopamine, which has a calming effect on the brain. As previously stated, any food rich in chlorophyll, such as the dark leafy greens, will provide plenty of magnesium.

Severe magnesium deficiencies have previously been considered to be uncommon in developed nations, because so many available foods contain magnesium. However, many people do not regularly get adequate magnesium from their diet, and it is now thought that up to 80 per cent of the population may be deficient in this mineral. A magnesium deficiency can have a profound impact on the functioning of the nervous system. Low levels of magnesium are associated with symptoms of anxiety, irritability, agitation insomnia and confusion, according to the University of Maryland Medical Centre. A review published in the December 1992 issue of the journal *Magnesium Research* reported that magnesium deficiency can result in neurological symptoms such as hyperexcitability, convulsions and a number of psychiatric symptoms, ranging from apathy to psychosis. Magnesium deficiency may also cause seizures. ME Morris, the author of the study, suggests that some of these symptoms may be reversed with magnesium supplementation.

Magnesium supplementation may help disorders associated with the nervous system. A study published in the October 2004 issue of the *Journal of the American College of Nutrition* reports that magnesium supplementation, combined with vitamin B-6, helped to correct symptoms of hyperexcitability, including aggression and inattention, in children. All 52 study participants experienced benefits from magnesium and vitamin B-6 treatment. A 2006 study in the journal *Medical Hypotheses* reported several case studies in which magnesium supplementation benefited patients suffering from 'major depression, traumatic brain injury, headache, suicidal tendencies, anxiety, irritability, insomnia, postpartum depression, cocaine, alcohol and tobacco abuse, hypersensitivity to calcium, short-term memory loss and IQ loss'.

That's a wide range of effects, indicating just how widespread this mineral is in its biochemical reactions.

The key with magnesium supplementation is to ensure that it is bioavailable (that is, that your body can absorb and make use of it). If you are not eating sufficient leafy greens, not drinking sufficient green juices and not using wheatgrass juice regularly, or have been shown to be deficient on blood testing, I suggest using a transdermal magnesium spray for best absorption.

The vitamin B12 issue

No discussion on the nervous system would be complete without a mention of the somewhat misnamed vitamin B12. B12 is not really a vitamin. It comes from a soil-based organism. It is still believed by many that vegans are the only population group that needs to consider B12 supplementation. However, recent research conducted by the Hippocrates Health Institute indicates that vitamin B12 deficiency is potentially a problem for 70 per cent of people, no matter what they eat, since many display problems with absorption of this essential nutrient, even if the dietary intake is adequate. Lack of hydrochloric acid in the stomach, as mentioned in chapter 2, will interfere with the absorption of B12.

Vitamin B12 works together with folate in the synthesis of DNA and red blood cells. It's also involved in the production of the myelin sheath (the insulating layer around the nerves, which protects the nerves and helps them to conduct messages). B12 has a range of actions in the body, and one of its most important functions in relation to the nervous system is in the prevention of brain shrinkage as we age. Given that the rates of dementia seem to be soaring in all developed countries, and also that B12 deficiency is known to produce a reversible dementia, it is high time we all took this bacteria-generated nutrient more seriously. Some studies have shown that not all dementia patients will respond to B12 supplementation. However, since supplementation seems to have a wide safety margin, I believe that it is a good starting point in anyone who is starting to display cognitive decline.

B12 supplementation is often necessary in people whose blood levels of the nutrient are within so-called 'normal' limits. Many clinicians believe that the lower end of the normal reference range is set too low; indeed, many people with so-called normal blood levels have demonstrated neurological disorders which respond to B12 supplementation. A better determination of our B12 status would be to measure the levels of methylmalonic acid (MMA) in the urine.

Tingling in the hands and feet, memory loss, learning disorders in children and depression/bipolar disorder can all be as a result of B12 deficiency, which thankfully responds to supplementation in most instances.

Of the types of supplementation available, Japanese studies indicate that methylcobalamin, as opposed to cyanocobalamin, is even more effective in treating the neurological consequences of B12 deficiency, and that it may be better absorbed because it bypasses several potential problems in the B12 absorption cycle. Additionally, methylcobalamin provides the body with methyl groups that play a part in various biological processes important to overall health (see also chapter 9).

I recommend that people use a soil-based form of vitamin B12 supplement (see the resources section at the end of this book).

Toxins that affect the nervous system

There are approximately 2000 new environmental chemicals that are produced each year, and many of these are created with little or no regulation. Released into the atmosphere, we come into contact with them through the air we breathe, the clothes we wear, the water we drink and the food we eat. Toxic metals are often considered to be the worst offenders, and affect not just the nervous system but also the endocrine system, liver, kidneys and immune system. An overview is given here since it is the nervous system that is most sensitive to these poisons.

Mercury

Mercury is the most toxic of all the metals, with the possible exception of uranium! It accumulates in the brain, heart, kidneys and endocrine glands and is responsible for diseases associated with 'demyelination' of the nerve sheaths – that is, the loss of the fatty covering of our nerve fibres, which enables efficient transmission of nerve impulses. Amalgam fillings, as mentioned in chapter 2, are 50 per cent mercury. According to the US Environmental Protection Agency, the mercury content from just one filling would create sufficient contamination to necessitate the closure of a 10-acre lake. We are exposed to mercury not just via fillings but also adhesives, air conditioning units, fabric softeners, floor wax, cosmetics, laxatives and tattoo ink, which also contains lead. Until very recently, mercury was used as a vaccine adjuvant. It is a deadly poison that causes brain damage (think of the 19th-century 'mad hatters' who used mercury to stiffen hats). More recently, mercury has been found to be present in large quantities in certain species of fish, as a result of environmental contamination of the seas. Fish is far from the health food that we are all being led to believe, and their contamination with deadly mercury is one of the chief reasons for this.

Lead

We are exposed to lead via older types of paint, insecticides, pottery, standard toothpaste, plastics, leaded petrol, batteries, newspaper, canned food and even chocolate, as reported by the National Institute of Environmental Health Science (Rankin CW, Nriagu JO, Flegal AR, 'Lead Contamination in Cocoa and Cocoa Products: Isotopic Evidence of Global Contamination', *Environmental Health Perspectives* 2005; 113(10): 1344-1348). Lead accumulates in the brain, bones, liver, kidneys and spleen. It alters behaviour and adversely affects intelligence.

Nickel

Nickel is present in cutlery, pots and pans, dental fillings and jewellery. It accumulates in bone, kidneys, sinuses, the brain and the immune system. Chronic nickel toxicity affects the skin.

Arsenic

Arsenic is present in cigarette smoke (along with 4000 other toxic chemicals), laundry detergent, beer, seafood, tap water, wine, synthetic-fibre clothes which are made from petrochemicals, plus those with 'easy-care' or 'non-iron' finishes, and older types of wallpaper. It accumulates in the liver, kidneys and lungs.

Cadmium

Cadmium is present in soft drinks, pesticides, fungicides, plastics, rustproofing, rubber, cigarette smoke and water softener. It accumulates in the kidneys, prostate and the eyes. A recent study indicated that 70 per cent of glaucoma patients had evidence of cadmium accumulation.

Uranium

A radioactive element, uranium causes cancer and birth defects. We all share one atmosphere. X-rays and CT scan usage has soared, and is now responsible for 50 per cent of the radiation that North Americans are exposed to – up from 15 per cent in 1980.

Aluminium

We are exposed to aluminium via water filtration units, deodorants, aluminium cans and fizzy drinks, and aluminium foil that food is wrapped in, as well as aluminium cooking utensils. It accumulates in bone, the kidneys and breast tissue. Underarm deodorants that contain aluminium increase the incidence of breast cancer. Aluminium contamination leads to stroke, heart attack and Alzheimer's disease.

Eliminating toxins

Toxic man-made debris and toxic metals can be difficult to eliminate from the body since they become incorporated into our very structure at a cellular level. Some of the metals mentioned above, at an atomic level, resemble familiar nutritional minerals and the body may try to use them as such: mercury can be mistaken for selenium, cadmium can be mistaken for zinc (we burn out zinc from the body when stressed, and zinc is essential for immunity), and aluminium, nickel and uranium can be mistaken for magnesium, which is also depleted if we are stressed.

Finally, it is important to mention that 80 per cent of baby products contain flame-retardant chemicals that cause cancer and brain damage. A study at Duke University revealed that car seats, high chairs and push chairs contain carcinogenic and mind-altering chemicals. All of these can be avoided.

A heavy metal detoxification regime can be used, which is described in my CD *The Importance of Detoxification*. This can safely be performed by anyone who is concerned about their toxic load. For anyone who is going to have amalgam fillings removed, this is essential. It's also a good idea to do this kind of detox regularly if you live in a polluted environment, such as a busy city.

In addition to toxic metals, it is also important to consider toxic chemicals in food which can affect the nervous system. These are mostly chemicals which are sprayed onto crops, and are therefore present in all conventionally grown, non-organic produce. Buy organic food wherever possible to avoid such chemicals, which can bio-accumulate in the body and are subsequently difficult to eliminate. Another emerging problem with agrochemicals is their potential to adversely affect the thyroid gland and act as a disruptive influence on the endocrine system, which I discuss in chapter 9.

Anyone for aspartame?

Described by some as the most dangerous chemical ever to enter the food chain, aspartame is an artificial sweetener that is 200 times as sweet as sugar. It is ubiquitously added to diet drinks and foods, and is present in approximately 5000 varieties of processed food. Passed by the American FDA (Food and Drug Administration) in a cloud of controversy in 1983, it has been linked to the following adverse effects, notably in connection with the nervous system:

Reduced vision	Reduced tear fluid production
Hearing impairment	Headaches
Dizziness	Mental confusion
Memory loss	Slurring of speech
Numbness and tingling of extremities	Tremors
Aggression	Depression and irritability
Insomnia	Anxiety
High blood pressure	Palpitations
Menstrual changes	Nausea
Excessive thirst	Weight gain
	Fluid retention and bloating
	...and even death.

Aspartame has no place in the human body, regardless of the purpose for which it was intended. Do not expose your nervous system to it, or any of your other systems for that matter. A safe, non-toxic sweetener for your food and drinks, if you feel that you need one, is stevia, a fine white powder which comes from the leaf of a plant and is becoming more widely accessible in health stores.

The mind-body connection

We can think our way to health and a calm nervous system. In the turmoil that many of us experience as daily life this can be challenging, but sitting calmly whilst repeating the following affirmations will help us to control all the negative 'mind-chatter' that may appear as a result of our perceived problems:

- I have faith that life is good and that I play an important part in it
- I have faith that good health is my natural birthright
- I have faith that the healing force within me will restore my health and strength, because I am the ultimate in- strument of my own healing
- I have faith that the universe and all of life assist me in my endeavours
- I am working positively toward harmony in and with all of life
- Harmony, strength and happiness are with me. I share them with all of life fully, openly, gratefully and joyfully.

Ultimately, the brain and nervous system control virtually everything in the body. We hear about the 'mind-body' con- nection all the time, and this is not just an unsubstantiated idea. Andy Bernay Roman states in his book *Deep Feeling, Deep Healing: The Heart, Mind and Soul of Getting Well* that the body follows what is in the heart and mind, which is being borne out through the emerging science of psychoneuroimmunology. In

Molecules of Emotion, Candace Pert relates that negative thoughts and stress actually have a physical structure in the body. This in turn can affect the way we carry ourselves. Look at the posture of a depressed person, for example. They are often slumped over, compressing their chest and restricting their breathing. Physiologically, if we smile we automatically produce chemical changes in the brain which make us feel happier. A fantastic teacher once told me that we should give everyone a smile in case they don't have one of their own.

One of the scientists whom I very much admire, Dr David Hamilton, says that we are all chemists. If we think about someone who makes us angry, we will produce stress hormones in the body. On the other hand, if we think about someone we love, or if we focus on compassion, we produce a 'love hormone' called oxytocin, which has some rather unusual properties. Used by vets as an injection to induce uterine contractions in animals, to assist the process of giving birth, oxytocin has other interesting physiological effects which are more far-reaching than we might imagine. It dilates the blood vessels, lowering the blood pressure, and has a protective effect on the heart. Oxytocin has also been shown to neutralise free radicals and reduce inflammation in the blood vessels. Not bad for something that you are just doing with your mind! David Hamilton also states that 'a hug a day keeps the cardiologist away', since hugs increase the secretion of oxytocin. Other benefits of focusing on love and compassion are that in addition to stimulating the production of oxytocin, you also increase secretions of the opioids serotonin and dopamine, the body's own version of morphine and heroin. No street drugs needed here – we have the power to create these chemicals just through focusing the mind.

Another fascinating effect of the nervous system can be seen by investigating the vagus nerve, which is the tenth cranial nerve. 'Vagus' means 'wanderer' and is so called because of its length and the fact that it wanders from the brainstem through the neck, chest and abdomen. Stimulation of the vagus nerve, also known as high vagal tone, gives better control of inflammation, and can also reduce epileptic seizures. Compassion has a stimulatory effect on the vagus nerve. The signal goes right down to our DNA and can turn on tumour necrosis factor (TNF-γ). The primary role of TNF is in the regulation of immune cells. TNF can induce death of cancer cells and prevent viral replication. Dysregulation of TNF production has been implicated in a variety of diseases, including Alzheimer's disease, cancer, major depression and inflammatory bowel disease. Dr Janet Hranicky, who runs her successful Cancer Reversal Program from the Hippocrates Health Institute, explains in her lectures how people can emotionally regulate their immune systems to increase the activity of natural killer (NK) cells, to attack and engulf cancer cells. How, therefore, can anyone possibly believe that the mind plays no part in health and well-being?

All of the above statements can be substantiated and measured. Via MRI scans, we can track the areas of the brain affected by different thought patterns, and relate, from that, what will happen physiologically. We have the ability, through blood samples, accurately to measure hormonal changes. We can evaluate the effects of stress on blood pressure, heart rate and body temperature. It is absolutely incredible what the mind can do, and we now know that by feeding our nervous system in a better way, ensuring it has the right fuel for its vast range of activities, we can influence the health of not just the nervous system, but in turn of all the other systems that it controls.

Could it be that the philosopher's stone and the elixir of life is actually internal? Perhaps we have never found it because we've been too busy looking *outside* the body!

A recipe for the nervous system: Romaine burritos

This recipe has been kindly contributed by Karen Ranzi, a living-foods teacher from the USA. With good levels of omega-3 fats and thiamine, Romaine lettuce contains some great nutrients for the nervous system, and the nuts used in the filling are high in good fats and magnesium.

Ingredients
One bunch large Romaine lettuce leaves

Taco flling
250 g (1 cup) of almonds or walnuts, soaked for 8-12 hours
125 ml (½ cup) lemon juice
60 g (¼ cup) sun-dried tomatoes, soaked for two hours, chopped
2 tablespoons chopped red onion
1 teaspoon each ground cumin, coriander and paprika
(can substitute 60 g / ¼ cup fresh cilantro for the ground coriander)

- Put all ingredients into a food processor with an S-blade.
- Process until smooth, or the consistency of a traditional bean dip is achieved.
- Add a little water if needed to get it moving.
- Add fresh tomato salsa on top for an extra taste treat.

Summary

- The nervous system is affected by food
- Blood sugar imbalances stress the nervous system
- Stress is damaging to the nervous system
- Green juice feeds the nervous system
- Vitamin B12 deficiency is harmful to the nervous system

- Magnesium is an essential nutrient for this system
- Meditation practice positively affects the brain
- The health of the mind determines the health of the whole body.

Chapter 6

The immune system

Fifty billion white blood cells working for you every day.

Some people go as far as to say that the immune system is by far your most important system. From my perspective, since we are only as strong as our weakest link, no one thing is more important than anything else. However, we only have to look at the devastation caused by the AIDS virus to know that without a correctly functioning immune system, life can get very difficult indeed.

The gut and immunity

One of the main benefits of the living foods lifestyle is the fantastic effect it has on rebuilding and rebalancing the immune system, and it is only a matter of time (and absorption of nutrients) before most people start to see and feel a difference. It is important to remember, as I stated in the chapter on intestinal function, that as much as 80 per cent of our immunity actually lies in our gut. Our probiotics colonise the lower digestive system, and if we have adequate numbers, we in fact have more bacterial cells than human cells in our bodies. The beneficial microflora are introduced at birth and are often topped up by eating dirt (it's actually natural for children to do this), but it is now often sadly depleted by frequent antibiotic usage and poor dietary choices, such as diets high in sugar, processed food and fat, which together provide unfavourable conditions for probiotic growth.

In the gut we have a vast network of lymphatic tissue known as the GALT (gut-associated lymphatic tissue) which constantly interfaces with our probiotic micro-organisms. This is essential for priming the immune system, teaching it to respond to bacteria without actually having to contract an infection – especially important for young children whose immune systems are not fully developed. When we hear of probiotics, many of us, as a result of aggressive marketing campaigns by dairy product manufacturers, tend to think of yogurt. However, you may be one of those who choose not to take dairy products in any form, as a result of the numerous problems associated with their consumption. The great news is that there are other ways to feed our microflora, with fermented food being the easiest. For those like me who dislike the taste of fermented food, a good-quality probiotic capsule is a simple alternative; I recommend Body Biotics, from Kiki Health (see resources).

Factors that affect immunity

Sleep

In our 24-hour society, it is often hard to get enough rest. Rest is essential for our immunity, and those of us who insist on burning the candle at both ends will eventually become ill, since fatigue and stress increase our susceptibility to disease, no matter what we eat. Stress is associated with increased secretion of cortisol and adrenaline. Cortisol suppresses the immune system and affects sugar metabolism, and regularly high levels are associated with obesity and the increased risk of infections. It is important to enjoy an active social life and have plenty of fun, but this should not be at the expense of adequate sleep.

Happiness and mood

Laughter genuinely could be considered to be the best medicine. In a recently published study in the journal *Alternative Therapies in Health and Medicine*, healthy women had a boost in their natural killer cell levels after watching funny videos, in comparison with those who watched a travel documentary. Getting together with friends and having a really good laugh should be high on the priority list of any health seeker. Indeed, having strong relationships and a good social network are vital for health.

Brian Clement, director of the Hippocrates Health Institute, states that psychotherapy and a positive attitude are the most beneficial things for the immune system, which he feels is 'God in action'. Most importantly, don't allow your healthy diet and lifestyle to make you feel like an outcast. John Robbins, in his wonderful book *Healthy at 100*, tells us that loneliness amongst the elderly has been shown to be a higher risk factor for death than smoking. Loneliness negatively affects the way in which some genes that control the immune system are expressed. Get involved with people in your community, regardless of what they eat. Join in, have fun and make a difference.

Sugar

High-sugar diets are a big concern with regard to the immune system. I go into a lot of detail on this subject in my CD *The Dangers of Excess Sugar Consumption*. For sure we all love a little indulgence, but basing any diet on cakes and indulgent desserts, raw or otherwise, could spell disaster for your immunity. Just because something is uncooked, it doesn't mean it's healthy! Eating foods high in sugar and fat reduces the ability of the white blood cells to overpower and destroy bacteria. This effect lasts several hours after consuming such foods. Consumption of sugar increases adrenaline production by 400 per cent, triggering our 'fear, fight, flight' mechanism and stressing the adrenals, as previously mentioned. If you're looking for a healthy sweetener to use in recipes, the best one is stevia, since it has no adverse effect on blood sugar regulation.

Exercise

Exercise is vital for the immune system, and I have already stated that 75 per cent of the potential benefits of the living foods lifestyle are lost if we don't exercise. There isn't always the incentive to exercise if it's cold and dark outside, but even getting your heart rate up for as little as 20 minutes, three or four times a week, has benefits, and studies show that a brisk walk five days a week reduces the risk of catching a cold, even for those on a standard diet. Exercise releases endorphins, the 'happy hormones' that improve sleep patterns and one's sense of well-being, both of which positively affect the immune system. Additionally, exercise is vital in the maintenance of ideal body weight. This has other benefits since studies show that not only does a high body fat level trigger the release of pro-inflammatory chemicals which damage the tissues, but also that obesity directly damages the immune system by reducing its antibody response.

Vitamin D

Low vitamin D levels are being shown to be harmful to the immune system, and new effects of the 'sunshine vitamin' are being discovered almost weekly. The active form of vitamin D is a hormone, produced in the skin upon exposure to ultraviolet light. Many North European vegans are deficient in vitamin D, since the sun is too low in the sky in winter to get any benefit from sunlight here, even if it were warm enough to expose the skin, which it is usually not. Many people do not get sufficient sun exposure in the summer and autumn to last them through the winter without supplementation, either with oral vitamin

D supplements or by taking a trip to the tropics. We know that vitamin D is important in bone health and the prevention of cancer, but it is also vital for the immune system, triggering and arming T cells, which seek out and destroy bacterial and viral invaders. Without sufficient vitamin D, T cells do not mobilise and remain dormant, according to scientists at the University of Copenhagen.

Since vitamin D is also significant in the expression of over 2000 genes (that is, only with sufficient vitamin D will you realise your full potential), I recommend having a blood test to check your levels of this vital hormone (25-OH D is the test to ask for; your GP should be able to do this test for you, or refer you to the relevant centre), and taking supplements of vitamin D3 if your levels prove to be low.

Garlic

Garlic is a true superfood not only for the circulation but also for the immune system. In addition to its phytonutrients ajoene and diallyl sulphide, which respectively prevent blood platelets from clumping and inhibit tumour formation, it contains allicin, which is a proven antibiotic. In moderate doses garlic inhibits more than 20 types of bacteria, at least 60 types of fungus and yeast, and in higher doses, eradicates them. Add fresh garlic cloves to your daily green juice or crush garlic onto your salads for a powerful cold and flu-fighting effect.

Antioxidants

Eating an antioxidant-rich diet is essential for immune function. We need to be aiming for a rainbow diet, incorporating as many different colours as possible, particularly the dark greens and purples. Fresh wheatgrass juice is a fantastic immune system booster and contains thousands of antioxidants. For additional antioxidant protection, ensure that your diet contains plenty of green sprouted food such as alfalfa, sunflower greens, sango radish, red clover, onion and broccoli.

I also recommend Juice Plus capsules (see appendix 2) for additional assistance with building the immune functions. The reason I recommend this particular product is because of the clinical trials that have been performed on it, not only with respect to the immune system (all parameters improved after 80 days on the capsules in one study), but also its bioavailability – that is, when you take it, it has been proven to get into the bloodstream where it is needed. This is my all-round supplement of choice and I have personally used it since 1995.

Prescription medicines

It is important to mention the effects of prescription medication in relation to the immune system. Antibiotic usage sadly leads us into a negative spiral – we have an infection because of a low immune function, we take antibiotics for that infection and the antibiotics cause further damage to the immune system, and so it goes on. To get out of this negative spiral, we need to work hard on all of the parameters that are known to be of benefit to the immune system. If we are faced with a life-threatening infection, then antibiotics can be essential. However, they are a short-term solution, and must be viewed as such. Antibiotic usage is known to damage the levels of probiotics in the gut, so if you have had a course of medication, ensure that you replace your probiotic organisms by eating fermented food or by taking a course of probiotics in capsule form.

Physical stimulation

Immune system functions have been shown to be improved by **cold water immersion**, and even by taking cold showers. Studies carried out in Prague have indicated that jumping into water at

14 °C, three times weekly, increases circulating levels of lymphocytes and monocytes, white blood cells which are involved in the immune response. In 1993, the UK's Thrombosis Research Institute reported that cold water activates the immune system by raising the metabolic rate. It's not just the immune system that benefits: NASA studies have shown that, over a 12-week period, repeated cold swimming leads to physiological changes known as cold adaptation. These bring down blood pressure and cholesterol, reduce fat deposition, inhibit blood clotting and increase fertility and libido in both men and women. The same benefits can be gained by showering. If you don't want the shock of getting straight into a cold shower, I suggest gradually turning the temperature down so that the body is not shocked. It has been suggested that alternate hot and cold showering can be very beneficial for the circulation too.

For those that like to pamper themselves, a **full body massage** is also of great benefit to the immune system, and not only from the perspective of stress reduction. Massage is known to reduce stress by increasing the production of oxytocin (see chapter 5, page 82), which in turn regulates the effects of stress hormones. Additionally, massage has also been shown to increase the production of cells that boost the immune system response, according to a recent study: Rapaport MH, Schettler P, Bresee C, 'A preliminary study of the effects of a single session of Swedish massage on hypothalamic-pituitary-adrenal and immune function in normal individuals', *The Journal of Alternative and Complementary Medicine* 2010; 16(10): 1–10.

Not every home will have one, and not everyone will have access to one, but a **far-infrared sauna** session has proven benefits for immunity. The heat produced in the sauna, and the penetration of the far-infrared rays below the skin surface, has a direct effect on the killing of pathogens, which cannot survive in the body above a certain critical temperature. The effect that raising the body temperature has on the immune system suggests that taking a sauna may help to fight infection and improve immune function. The improved immune function that occurs with the activation of white blood cells together with increases in important immune signals and proteins, in addition to the direct effect of elevated temperature on bacteria and viruses, make the sauna a safe adjunctive therapy for infections and possibly allergies. The relaxed feeling one gets from a sauna session is also beneficial in stress reduction, in turn essential for boosting immunity.

Getting out in nature is now being recommended by Japanese scientists as a way of boosting the immune system. They are even suggesting that getting lost in the woods can be good for you from the perspective of enhanced immunity, provided that the process of getting lost doesn't stress you out, of course. Unlikely as it might appear, **drumming sessions** are also stated to boost immunity. A recent medical research study indicated that drumming circles have beneficial effects for the immune system. Led by renowned cancer expert Barry Bittman, MD, the study demonstrated that group drumming increases cancer-killing cells, which help the body combat not just cancer but also certain viruses, including AIDS. According to Dr Bittman, 'Group drumming tunes our biology, orchestrates our immunity, and enables healing to begin.'

A recipe for the immune system: Middle Eastern salad

This recipe comes courtesy of Judy Barber, (www.judy-barber. com), author of *Good Raw Food Recipes*, a highly recommended book. Judy explains below why this recipe is great for your immune system. Thank you, Judy.

'Dark green vegetables are wonderful for immune system support, as in this mild green salad with a spiced dressing featuring the Middle Eastern spice "sumac", the crushed dried berries of the sumac tree. I happily discovered sumac when living in Iran, where it is served as a condiment in roadside cafes. It has a sour, slightly lemony flavour and a particularly high ORAC value [ORAC is an acronym for "oxygen radical absorption capacity", and is a measurement of the ability of a food to scavenge harmful free radicals. High ORAC value foods are loaded with antioxidants]. Find it in an Asian delicatessen or online. The cumin, turmeric, cayenne, lemon and garlic nourish and boost the immune system, the garlic having antibacterial and antiviral properties. Until you track down the sumac, try making this with a tablespoon of lemon juice instead. Rough quantities below are for two to four people.

Ingredients
4 big handfuls of spinach leaves
$^2/_3$ of a cucumber
2 handfuls of pea shoots and/or homegrown sunflower greens
60 ml (¼ cup) cold pressed virgin olive oil
½ a small ripe lemon
1 heaped teaspoon sumac powder, plus more in a small dish to serve alongside
1 small piece of garlic, crushed
½ teaspoon cumin powder
1 pinch cayenne
2 teaspoons tamari soya sauce

- Wash the spinach and slice finely.
- Slice the cucumber finely in rounds or short thin trips and arrange or mix the salad in a bowl.
- Slice the lemon, skin and all, and chop finely. Sprinkle over the salad.
- Mix the oil, spices, garlic and tamari. Drizzle over the salad or serve alongside.

Summary

- Much of your immune system lies in your gut
- Probiotics are important
- High-sugar diets damage the immune system
- Stress negatively affects this system via the action of cortisol
- Certain whole-food supplements have proven benefits for immunity
- Vitamin D is essential for a strong immune system
- Far-infrared saunas boost immunity
- A massage can help your immune system.

Chapter 7

The respiratory system

The surface of a tennis court, with 1600 km of blood vessels – how does all that fit into your chest?

There is nothing better than a big breath of fresh air. We all know how much better we feel when breathing in clear, unpolluted mountain air. Ever wondered why? The respiratory system provides oxygen to the cells. Without oxygen our cells rapidly malfunction and die. We can survive weeks without food, days without water, but only minutes without air.

The upper part of the system – mouth, nose, sinuses, and larynx – help filter, humidify and warm the air as it enters the body. The little hair-like structures (cilia) in the lining of our air passages, and the mucus, protect our lungs from dirt and dust. The air travels through the increasingly narrow passages of our respiratory system – the trachea, bronchi and bronchioles – and finally into the alveoli, the thousands of minute sacs where gaseous exchange takes place. Oxygen from the air then passes into the blood and on to the heart, and in turn through the circulatory system to oxygenate the cells. On exhalation, the blood carries the carbon dioxide and other wastes into the alveoli, to go back out through the lungs, trachea and finally out via the mouth or nose.

Ways to maintain a healthy respiratory system

The following will help to maintain a healthy respiratory system:

- Practise deep abdominal breathing. Deep breathing in nature is excellent for the respiratory system. Yoga practice is also very good for the lungs.
- **Exercise**, especially outside in fresh air. Physical exercise strengthens the muscles as well as the muscles of the diaphragm. It relaxes the body, increasing blood circulation. The body is better able to eliminate waste and toxic materials more quickly, allowing the body to benefit from better-quality oxygen. Vigorous exercise is excellent, or in fact, when just starting, even moderate exercise. Anything is better than nothing.
- **Breathe fresh air** as much as possible. Make sure your house is well ventilated, not too dry or too humid, and that your heating/cooling system is clean. Switching to 'green' cleaning products will also improve indoor air quality.
- Drink plenty of pure **water**.
- Eat a **healthy diet**, free from dairy products. In particular, the following foods nourish the respiratory system:

Garlic	Onions
Leeks	Turnip
Grapes	Pineapple
Dark leafy greens	Fresh vegetable juices
Carrots	Watercress
Apples	

- **Eliminate regularly**. We need to have two or more bowel movements per day and maintain a healthy intestinal flora.
- **Reduce acidity** in the body by eliminating processed food, caffeine and alcohol.
- **Never smoke**, or expose yourself to passive smoking.
- Avoid foods that increase mucus in the body (see below).

The problem with mucus

Many of my clients mention in their lifestyle analysis forms that they have problems with excess mucus; dairy products are a major cause of difficulty in this regard. The main problem with dairy products is that after age three years we gradually lose the capacity to break them down fully, especially if they are cooked and come from the wrong species of mammal in the first place. As adults, often the best we can do is break down dairy products into a compound called a dipeptide, which consists of two amino acids joined together. These are small enough to pass into the blood stream, but are not recognisable as individual amino acids, so they elicit an immune response. To eliminate them, they are often pushed out through the mucous membrane of the respiratory system, damaging it and allowing the appearance of a 'cold'. This is not really a cold, of course. For infection to occur, we have to have a pathogenic bacterium or virus, something for that bug to feed on (dairy produce is ideal for this) and a damaged mucous membrane (which is damaged by trying to eliminate said dairy produce).

Many young children and even some adults undergo tonsillectomy as a cure for permanently inflamed tonsils or the appearance of regular bouts of tonsillitis. I personally underwent this procedure in 1969; I am convinced that in my case the underlying cause of all my problems was an immune reaction to incompletely digested, pasteurised dairy produce, and nothing to do with 'true' infection. Unfortunately for me, my doctor did not believe that allergies existed and my parents trusted and followed the recommendations that he put forward. For anyone considering tonsillectomy for their child, my personal recommendation would be first to eliminate dairy products from his or her diet to see if the condition clears up. If it does not, then by all means continue with surgery, but it is always worth trying a more natural, diet-oriented approach first for this distressing but non-life-threatening condition.

Foods that increase mucus

Foods that increase mucus in the body are unhealthy for all the body systems, especially the respiratory system. These include:

- Refined sugar
- Dairy products, especially when pasteurised
- White foods, such as sugar, flour, white rice
- All refined, processed foods
- Additives and food colouring
- Concentrated fruit juices
- Too many fruits.

The body produces mucus to protect itself. When there are too many toxins invading the body, excess mucus is produced, first in the digestive system and then in other organs, especially the respiratory system. Excess mucus accumulates in the sinuses, bronchioles, throat and lungs. The tonsils and ears are also frequently affected.

What was a defence system for the body now becomes a barrier, preventing the passage of nutrients and oxygen. This results in a myriad of diseases. Of course cigarette smoke and pollution play an important part in respiratory illnesses, but a healthy diet is of utmost importance.

Signs of excess mucus in the body include:

- Recurring sinus infections
- Nasal drip
- Hay fever and allergies
- Persistent cough and hoarse throat
- Digestive problems
- Constipation or diarrhoea
- Burping, gas
- Bad breath
- Asthma and respiratory problems

- Excess wax build-up in ears, itchy eyes
- Polyps, tumours
- Feeling discouraged, tired, unhappy.

Asthma

An estimated 300 million people worldwide suffer from asthma, and asthma has increased 75 per cent since 1980. Our respiratory systems therefore need all the help they can get. There is so much you can do to treat asthma naturally, and cleaning up the diet and the home environment are great places to start. The diet that helps all the other body systems is also one that will allow asthmatics to heal naturally. Here are some foods that are known to aggravate asthma; interestingly, several on this list are the very same foods that can cause problems with digestion, brain function, immunity and hormonal balance:

- Dairy produce
- White refined sugar
- White flour
- Gluten
- Table salt
- Processed foods
- Foods containing artificial colours and other additives
- Peanuts
- Corn
- Colas and other canned fizzy drinks
- Soya.

Conclusion

There is a lot that you can do to alleviate or completely clear up respiratory ailments. The first step is in making changes in your diet to ensure you are getting the proper nutrients your body needs. Eliminate all dairy products and foods mentioned above that could be aggravating the condition.

Finally, and probably most importantly of all, excessive stress will impact the respiratory system since it shifts the breathing patterns from slow, deep, abdominal breathing to short, shallow, more 'clavicular' breathing, coming from the upper chest. Another good reason to get on with the meditation practice...

A recipe for the respiratory system: Root veggies pâté

This recipe was contributed by Karen Ranzi, MA, a raw vegan chef and director of www.superhealthychildren.com. Karen found the natural path that enabled her son to heal from asthma, chronic ear infections and multiple food allergies in 1994. By means of her education, life-changing personal experiences and sincere desire to share her message, Karen has been able to guide thousands of families toward developing excellent health.

Karen has included rutabaga (swede) in this recipe for its multiple health benefits, notably its benefits for bronchitis.

Ingredients
3 medium carrots, chopped
1 stalk celery, chopped
1 medium rutabaga, peeled and chopped
Juice of ½ lemon
Juice of ½ lime
2 tablespoons of raw tahini (sesame seed paste)

- Process carrots, celery and rutabaga in food processor until finely ground.
- Add lemon and lime juice and tahini and process until a smooth pâté.
- This is one of my favourite dishes to place over a large green salad for a complete meal. I find it to be especially satisfying during the cold winter months.
- Variation: I love dill and sometimes add 2 tablespoons of dill to this tasty recipe.

Summary

- Exercise is essential for good lung function
- Indoor and outdoor air pollution harms the respiratory system
- Mucus-forming foods should be avoided
- Stress can be detrimental to this system
- Look for green cleaning products
- Get outside in nature whenever you can.

Chapter 8

The urinary system

One to two million nephrons per kidney, and 50 litres of blood per hour.

Your urinary system includes your kidneys, bladder, ureters and urethra. Its job is to filter and eliminate waste products from your blood stream and to help regulate fluid and salt balance in your food. Unlike many of the other internal organs, the kidneys cannot regenerate. They can be damaged by high-protein diets, such as the Atkins diet, the Zone diet and the Sugar Buster diet. This damage occurs only when eating high levels of animal protein, not plant protein; another good reason never to eat meat.

Water

The urinary system is the body's water regulator. One of the benefits of moving to a raw diet is that organic water, which is lost during cooking, is preserved. However, we still need to drink. The large green juice (see page 19) daily will improve hydration at a cellular level, and allow the kidneys to function better. In addition to this, I recommend drinking about 1.5 to 2 litres of pure filtered water every day. If your urine is clear and you are urinating 10 to 12 times a day that's about right. At the Hippocrates Health Institute it has been calculated that you need to drink half a fluid ounce of water per pound of bodyweight per day, so work out what that means for you and aim to reach that daily target. However, don't drink tap water whatever you do.

As you may have already picked up from earlier chapters, I am not a fan of drinking municipal water straight out of the tap. The main reason is that it contains chlorine, which is linked to a stack of potential health concerns. Studies conducted as long as 20 years ago indicate that chlorinated drinking water predisposes us to atherosclerotic plaque, something that I discuss in relation to the circulatory system (see page 55). There are many other options for how we can obtain clean and pure water, but having said that I don't recommend tap water, I have to say that I don't recommend bottled water either.

Bottled water is immensely draining on natural resources, with the plastic bottles accounting for the use of more than 15 million barrels of oil annually. Moreover, the bottles are generally blown at the springs that the water comes from. This in itself would not be problematic if they were allowed to cool to the extent that no plastic leakage would occur into the water. This, sadly, does not appear to be the case, and the water in these bottles contains leached plastic. This can have a detrimental effect on the body since the plastic comes from petrochemicals, and plastic in our system acts as a xenoestrogen – an oestrogen-mimicking chemical which creates havoc with our natural hormonal balance (see chapter 9). Pure water can definitely be obtained from a natural spring, but you would need to store it in glass bottles, or hard plastic bottles that are free from Bisphenol-A (BPA), a chemical which is considered by toxicologists to be a disrupter of endocrine function. In 2008 the National Toxicology Program, part of the USA's National Institute of Health, expressed concern that BPA affects the prostate gland, the brain and the development of fetuses, infants and children. BPA's detrimental effects aren't just confined to the hormonal system. They are also a cause of oxidative stress, which as we know from previous chapters adversely affects the immune system and accelerates ageing. The good news is that wheatgrass juice appears to counteract this damage (Yi B, Kasai H, Lee HS, Kang Y, Park JY, Yang M, 'Inhibition by wheat sprout (Triticum aestivum) juice of Bisphenol A-induced oxidative stress in young women', *Mutation Research* 2011; 724(1-2): 64-88), but BPA is still best avoided.

A more simple method of ensuring better quality water in the home is to filter it. The most commonly used type of filtration system is a granular activated carbon system, generally with silver. These filters remove the chlorine and particulate material, and need to be replaced periodically to ensure that they remain bacteriostatic (able to inhibit the multiplication of bacteria) – generally, every three years. Reverse osmosis machines incorporate two types of water purification – filtration and reverse osmosis, whereby the water is forced under pressure through a semi-permeable membrane which is able to reduce inorganic minerals. This system can remove up to 90 per cent of mineral, organic and biological contaminants.

Water distillation removes more contaminants – 99.9 per cent of them to be precise. There is some controversy about drinking distilled water. Some authors, for example Brian Clement from the Hippocrates Institute, state that it is the best thing for us to do, whilst others, such as Dr Zoltan Rona, submit that it is an 'aggressive' form of water and has no place in our bodies. I side with the former argument; we know that inorganic minerals in the drinking water accumulate in the body and are not incorporated as beneficial nutrients.

The latest form of water purification device is the newer technology of atmospheric water generation. This extracts water directly from the air, in the same way that a room dehumidifier would. This bypasses all of the contaminants that are likely to be found in the municipal water supply, and for example lead supply pipes in older houses. After extraction from the air, the water is passed through a multi-stage filtration and other treatment processes, giving 99.9 per cent purity.

Whichever way we choose to purify our water, there is a lot that can be done to 'restructure' it afterwards. Previously considered to be on the outer edges of science, there are now many studies that indicate that water is a particularly unique type of fluid with some unusual properties, and can take on the memory of substances which have been dissolved in it. Also, if we study the independent work of Masaru Emoto and Viktor Schauberger, we find that water can be imprinted with the emotions of how we think and feel, and the way in which water flows can have either a health-enhancing or health detracting effect. Emoto's books include *The Hidden Messages in Water* and *The True Power of Water*, both of which make a fascinating read.

Be aware that tea and coffee are dehydrating to the body, as is alcohol. I have heard it stated that they all have benefits for the body's fluid balance, but remain unconvinced of this since they are all diuretics. Eliminate coffee and standard tea. Even green tea contains caffeine, but if you feel you need to use green tea as you transition off normal tea and coffee, then go ahead. Ideally, no caffeine should be consumed since it is highly irritating to the nerves and adrenal glands. Whatever you do, do not use decaffeinated drinks. They usually still contain quite a lot of caffeine, even if labelled decaffeinated, and the decaffeination process involves turpentine and embalming fluid, neither of which we want in the body.

Food for the urinary system

A healthy diet provides your urinary system with nutrients it requires to function efficiently. Certain foods offer particularly high levels of urinary-health-boosting benefits.

Berries

Berries may promote urinary tract health and provide protection against infection, according to the *Harvard Medical School Family Health Guide*. Flavonols in berries, the compounds plants use to fight bacterial infections, may be responsible for the benefits seen in humans. A glass of berry juice once a day may reduce your risk of developing a urinary tract infection by up to 34 per cent. One study, reported in the *Journal of Medicinal Food*, found that cranberry juice prevents bacteria from sticking to the lining of the urinary tract, thereby lowering infection risk. The effects of the cranberry juice continued to increase for at least eight hours. If considering cranberry juice, bear in mind that many processed and packaged juices contain a large quantity of added sugar, and sugar in any quantity detracts from urinary health. Adding fresh cranberries to a green juice would be a better option in my opinion.

Garlic

Garlic exhibited potential benefits against bladder cancer in a tissue-culture study published in the January-February 2011 issue of the journal *Molecular Medicine Reports*. Garlic extract induced cell death in bladder cancer cells and inhibited cancer cells from migrating and metastasising. Researchers concluded that garlic may offer potential benefits in the treatment and prevention of bladder cancer. Garlic also shows possible protective effects for the kidneys, according to a laboratory animal study on chronic kidney failure published in 2011 (Deniz M, Şener G, Ercan F, Yeğen BÇ, 'Garlic extract ameliorates renal and cardiopulmonary injury in the rats with chronic renal failure', *Renal Failure* 2011; 33(7): 718-725). Supplementation with garlic for three weeks reduced inflammation and decreased white blood cell levels.

Antioxidants

Proanthocyanidin antioxidants in apples, grapes, peanuts and cinnamon may help maintain the health of the urinary tract, whilst grape seed extract, obtained from grape juice or by eating grapes with seeds, may prevent kidney disease by prolonging the life of kidney cells and protecting against oxidation, according to a recent study (Ulusoy S, Ozkan G, Yucesan FB, Ersöz Ş, Orem A, Alkanat M, Yuluğ E, Kaynar K, 'Anti-apoptotic and anti-oxidant effects of grape seed proanthocyanidin extract in preventing cyclosporine A-induced nephropathy', *Nephrology* (Carlton). 2012; 17(4): 372-379).

A recipe for the urinary system: Cranberry and coconut juice

Ingredients
150 g (¾ cup) fresh cranberries, juiced
Water from two fresh coconuts, or one 250 ml carton of unpasteurised coconut water
2 ice cubes

- Combine the freshly juiced cranberries with the coconut water, add ice cubes and enjoy as a refreshing, hydrating drink.

Summary

- Excess animal protein consumption can damage the kidneys
- Filtering your drinking water is essential to remove contaminants
- Restructuring your drinking water is recommended
- Diuretic drinks, such as coffee and alcohol, cause the kidneys to eliminate more water and so cause dehydration.

Chapter 9

The hormonal system

Over 30 hormones, affecting sleep, sex and happiness...

This chapter looks at the main hormonal systems of the body, and the profound impact that our food and lifestyles can have on their levels, both beneficially and otherwise. I'm going to start off by diving straight into the sex hormones, and discussing exactly how imbalances here can have wide-reaching effects on our bodies, and what we need to do about it.

Sex hormones and the problem of oestrogen dominance

One of the growing concerns about our hormonal health in recent years has come from the many conditions that are all closely related to oestrogen dominance (an imbalance, notably excess, of oestrogen in relation to the other sex hormones), leaving us immunologically susceptible to such conditions as syndrome X, diabetes and cancer as we age. Oestrogen dominance, first described by Dr John R Lee in his book *What your doctor may not tell you about menopause* (Warner Books, 1996), is becoming increasingly common in the developed world. It has a detrimental effect on levels of thyroid hormone, progesterone, vitamin D3, testosterone and DHEA (dehydroepiandrosterone, a precursor to both male and female sex hormones) in both men and women. Our sex hormones are fundamentally signallers, and whilst a surge of oestradiol is appropriate in girls of age 14, it is definitely not desirable at the age of 65, since at this life-stage it would drive the development of abnormal cells in breast tissue. Conversely, progesterone signalling improves immunity, is anti-ageing, improves lean muscle mass and reduces fat storage, which is a far more desirable outcome. Cortisol, whilst not specifically a sex hormone, can have similar effects to oestrogen dominance, when it is out of balance.

Birth control pills cause oestrogen dominance, which is a huge concern given how widespread their use is. I know of very few women who have never taken such prescriptions, and I always think how sad that is, to have so many people not knowing the compounding harm they are causing themselves in the long term. In addition to certain foods being oestrogenic, such as soya, most of the commonly used pesticides also act as oestrogen mimickers. This is a bad thing if you happen to live near a large-scale commercial farm that is liberally spraying pesticides on crops, and also a very good reason to eat organic food.

We may have heard from health journalists about xenoestrogens – oestrogen-mimicking hormones that come from leached plastics and cause mayhem, disrupting the delicate balance of our natural oestrogens. Xenoestrogens are not only taken in orally but can gain access to the body via the skin. Brian Clement, in his book *Killer Clothes*, warns that many man-made fibres that are produced from petrochemicals are xenoestrogenic. This is a good reason to ensure that you give priority to choosing clothes that are made from natural fibres rather than synthetic. When phytoestrogenic compounds are taken in through food, we at least stand a chance of detoxifying them via the liver's activity of methylation (adding a 'methyl group' compound which is part of the detoxification process). However, xenoestrogens absorbed through the skin get straight into the bloodstream, so the liver does not have a chance of detoxifying these chemicals. Over time, oestrogen-mimickers in the liver cause age-related problems if their detoxification is not performed adequately.

The so-called 'bad oestrogens', which the body produces itself, have a chemical structure that is non-methylated (that is, they do not contain a methyl group, as described above, as part of their chemical structure). By consuming foods that are 'methyl group donors', we can detoxify these dangerous compounds more readily so that they don't wreak havoc in our body. Methyl group donors are useful in other respects; homocysteine, which together with CRP (C-reactive protein) is strongly implicated in heart disease, ageing and the risk of stroke, is an amino acid which is non-methylated and therefore detoxified more readily in the presence of methyl group donors.

The best foods and compounds that act as **methyl group donors** are as follows:

- Beetroot (both raw and fermented)
- Goji berries
- MSM (see chapter 10)
- SAMe (S-adenosyl methionine, a food supplement used for liver support)
- Vitamins B6, B9 and B12.

We have three types of oestrogen in the body (oestriol, oestradiol and oestrone), and when having blood tests done it is useful to know which ones may be out of balance, so testing for all three types is important. Oestrone is the most problematic, followed by oestradiol. Oestriol is considered to be the safest type of oestrogen. According to David Wolfe, from a presentation given at the Women's Wellness Conference in early 2013, nutritional compounds present in lemon and lime rind dissolve bad oestrogen. He also states that as a bonus, using lemon and lime rind in juices helps to eliminate cellulite, which he believes is an accumulation of bad oestrogen together with calcification of the tissues. No wonder he's so popular with the ladies.

Iodine, which is well known to feed the thyroid tissue, is also important in protection against bad oestrogen. Dietary fibre is essential in binding unwanted oestrogen and assisting its removal from the body. In addition to fibre, the following foods also possess phytonutrients that are important in blocking the adverse effects of oestrogenic compounds:

- Berries
- Broccoli (especially broccoli sprouts)
- Kale
- Green tea (but remember, it contains caffeine)
- Defatted flax
- Sesame seeds
- Apples
- Mushrooms.

Some words about HRT

Many women experience an early or an uncomfortable meno-pause. Interestingly, the Japanese language has no word for the somewhat Western condition of 'hot flush'. The almost instant reaction of the medical profession to this distressing female con-dition still seems to be to reach for hormone replacement, often, shockingly, without even evaluating what the pre-existing levels of the individual sex hormones are in each woman.

A case in point is that of a work colleague of mine, who, as a result of persistent headaches, was put onto HRT, because she is of a 'certain age'. HRT is of course in itself not particularly horrifying. After all, it is very common for it to be prescribed to women. What I found disturbing about the particular case of my work colleague was the fact that the treatment had just been prescribed 'blind'. I asked her which of her hormones had been shown to be low on her blood tests. Her reply was, 'I didn't have any blood tests; they just put me on the HRT.'

Recently, the BMA (British Medical Association) issued a

statement that the use of HRT is now considered to be far less necessary than was originally thought, and that every potential recipient should be assessed on a 'risk to reward' basis, since the adverse effects of 'supplementing' with hormones are well known. It would appear that this information had not yet filtered down to my colleague's doctor, or indeed to the doctors of many of my other clients who have been prescribed these potentially hazardous chemicals. The side effects include bleeding, thrombus (blood clot) formation, breast cancer, endometriosis, stroke, uterine cancer and more.

I then questioned my colleague further. Which hormones had she been put on, and were they a bioidentical type, or synthetic? She confessed that she didn't actually know, and was surprised to learn that there was a difference between the two.

Why should I be horrified by this situation? Firstly, HRT has become so widely accepted that peri- and post-menopausal women have been brainwashed into thinking that it is good for them. Consequently, they rarely feel the need to question its relevance in their individual situation. Secondly, the differences between synthetic and bio-identical hormones are not being adequately explained to patients, though this will affect whether any dangerous side effects of the medication are experienced. However, what disturbs me most about this particular story is that no blood tests were taken to establish whether my colleague's symptoms were the result of a hormonal irregularity. Surely this has to be questioned? How can anyone possibly know what is happening in someone else's body without the vital information that blood tests reveal? What if the headaches were due to stress or dehydration, or poor diet, or a myriad of other possibilities? Were these possibilities considered? Were they investigated? And, dare I ask, was the doctor male or female?

HRT is not confined to women. Men can exhibit andropause, and experience increased body fat, mood changes and even the development of breasts.

There are six sex hormones that need to be evaluated before anyone, in my opinion, should ever allow HRT to be used. These are oestradiol, oestriol, oestrone, DHEA, progesterone and testosterone. If any of these are deficient, the supplementation should be with the spectrum of those that are low, not just one or two of them. And you should never, ever, allow synthetic hormones into your body. Only the natural, bioidentical type should be used. It may mean that you have to go to see a clinician who specialises in this type of sex hormone endocrinology. If that is the case, do it. Your body is far too valuable to allow anyone to treat it 'blind'.

It is also now recommended that anyone on HRT should be evaluated annually. I go into further detail in my book *Top 10 Raw Food Tips for Osteoporosis* on the six sex hormones and how their levels affect us, mainly in relation to bone health. However, I also emphasise the importance of ensuring that only bio-identical hormones are used and that blood tests are carried out to assess the need for them in the first place. If you are currently receiving HRT and have not recently had an evaluation of your unique requirement for it, I recommend that you do so.

The pancreas

The pancreas produces two major hormones that regulate blood sugar: insulin and glucagon. The incidence of adult onset (type 2) diabetes is now becoming so common that it is worthy of special comment here.

The challenges associated with diabetes are immense. In a report published after an audit of UK patients in 2011, it was announced that the NHS faces a 'diabetes time bomb', with 800,000 people having elevated blood sugar which could lead to kidney failure, limb amputation and stroke. This report came at about the same time that other news stories indicated that diabetes rates worldwide had doubled within a short time frame. Despite some authors still being convinced that there is a genetic basis for type 2 diabetes, we know that type 2, or insulin resistance, can be totally reversed with dietary change and exercise. Gabriel Cousens demonstrates in his book *There is a Cure for Diabetes* that by adopting a living foods regime the disease can be reversed in as little as 30 days. Reports from the Hippocrates Health Institute show similar findings with insulin resistance.

Type 1 diabetes is less easy to control. Adopting a living foods lifestyle is only about 30 per cent effective in reversing the condition. However, up to 70 per cent of those affected by type 1 are able dramatically to reduce their insulin dose by adopting a living foods lifestyle. Type 1 diabetes is more a matter of prevention. We know that the condition is caused by a progressive destruction of the beta cells in the 'islets of Langerhans' in the pancreas, and it is noteworthy that juvenile (type 1) diabetes is 36 times more common in Finland than it is in Japan. The main difference between the diets of young Finns and young Japanese is the presence of large quantities of dairy products in diets in Finland. The way pasteurised dairy products, in particular, seem to coat the pancreatic cells is one of the main considerations in the development of the condition. Immune complexes triggered by either bovine serum albumin or bovine insulin could also be contributing factors.

A counter-argument to these findings, unsurprisingly put forward by the dairy industry, states that this is not the case, or could only be the case if the child is already genetically predisposed to type 1 diabetes. However, we know that bad genes can be suppressed indefinitely through good nutrition and lifestyle factors, so the advice here would be to breastfeed as long as possible, and to use raw goat's milk for children up to age three. After this age, children no longer need a dietary source of cholesterol, so milk products in any form are no longer necessary, and should not be part of the diet.

We can read any number of frightening statistics regarding diabetes, fast becoming one of our major killers, but the fact remains that, the condition doesn't stand a chance against people armed with an excellent living foods diet and a willingness to exercise.

Leptin and fructose

It is worth mentioning a little about **leptin** here, and the problems associated with the consumption of **fructose**, the sugar predominantly found in fruit. Have you ever been in the position of being constantly hungry no matter what you ate, as if a switch in your brain had been turned on and you weren't able to find the off switch? The problem could well be related to your fructose intake. Manufactured primarily in fat cells, leptin is one of the main hormones that informs the body whether food intake is needed. On eating, leptin levels increase, signalling to the appetite centre in the hypothalamus that you have eaten and need no further intake. Leptin inhibits the appetite to prevent overeating. If leptin levels are low, people will be more likely to have a higher caloric intake and therefore gain weight, according to a June 2004 paper published in the *Journal of Clinical Endocrinology & Metabolism*.

Because insulin and leptin function as key signals to the central nervous system in the long-term regulation of energy balance, reduced circulating insulin and leptin could lead to increased caloric intake, and ultimately contribute to weight gain and obesity during chronic consumption of diets high in fructose.

The challenge that we have in the developed world is that fructose is everywhere! All processed foods contain it, and it is being added to food in vast quantities in the form of high-fructose corn syrup. High-fructose corn syrup is less than half the price of sugar, and has been added to practically everything that is processed, from fast food to ready meals. It is ubiquitous in fizzy drinks and all colas, as well as fruit drinks and cordials. The raw food world has not escaped its clutches. Agave syrup, purported to be a healthy sweetener by many, is as bad as high-fructose corn syrup. Much dried fruit is high in fructose, particularly dates and figs. The only individuals who should ever consider eating dried fruit, in my opinion, are high-performance athletes. A process known as 'glycation', the joining of fructose or glucose to protein, predisposes to the generation of free radicals, which are accelerators of all disease processes and ageing. The research is irrefutable: if your aim is to be obese and experience rapid ageing and degeneration, a high-fructose diet is the fastest way to achieve this.

The thyroid gland

The paired thyroid glands lie in the middle of the neck, either side of the trachea (windpipe), and in close proximity to some other important anatomical structures, namely the jugular vein, carotid artery, recurrent laryngeal nerve and the parathyroid glands. The thyroid is considered by many to be the master gland of metabolism, since underactivity leads to a slowed metabolism, weight gain, lethargy and other undesirable characteristics. The two main hormones produced by the thyroid gland are thyroxine (T4) and tri-iodothyronine (T3). You can probably work out, by the name for the thyroid hormone, T3, that it has iodine in its structure, and, unsurprisingly, good levels of iodine are necessary for the correct functioning of the thyroid gland. Seaweed is a useful food for most people, which because of its iodine content, feeds the thyroid. However, high levels of dietary iodine can be contraindicated in certain medical conditions, such as, for example, Hashimoto's thyroiditis, an autoimmune condition. I have found conflicting arguments both for and against its use in Hashimoto's, so if you have this particular condition, check with your doctor first before suddenly eating a lot of seaweed.

The recommended quantity of seaweed to eat per day is between 15 and 25 grams. This doesn't sound like a lot, but dried seaweed is incredibly light, so it actually can look like quite a lot on the plate. Not only does seaweed give the body the necessary iodine levels to ensure that you can manufacture adequate levels of thyroid hormone, it also provides numerous other important minerals for our structural systems, especially the hair, skin and nails.

Another excellent food for the thyroid gland is coconut oil. In the health literature you will find that some authors devote whole books to the many health benefits of coconut oil, even to the point at which they imply that it cures every ailment known to man. On the other hand, you will find others who state that more than a tablespoon a day of coconut oil can cause your blood cholesterol levels to rise, even though the coconut oil itself contains no cholesterol. As always, common sense should prevail. My suggestion would be to limit your consumption to two teaspoons daily for thyroid health. More is not always better.

More nutrients for your thyroid

Like every cell and organ in our bodies, the thyroid requires specific vitamins and minerals to carry out everyday functions. Though there are many nutrients the thyroid uses, I'll highlight those that research shows to be most crucial. We've evolved to extract these micronutrients from the foods we eat (see below for raw plant foods you can eat to obtain these nutrients). You may also choose to supplement, but before starting any supplements for thyroid function, I encourage you to learn more about your individual needs. If you think you may have a thyroid imbalance, it's a good idea to see a healthcare practitioner to request a full thyroid hormone profile, as well as to have your iodine, selenium and vitamin D levels tested. Most functional medicine practitioners are familiar with this style of testing.

Iodine

Your thyroid simply cannot function without this crucial trace element, and if you are iodine-deficient, higher iodine intake could make all the difference to your thyroid. The essential thyroid hormones that circulate in our bodies, known, as already mentioned, as T4 (also called 'thyroxine') and the more active T3, are the only iodine-containing hormones in humans. According to a 2012 report by the Centers for Disease Control and Prevention (CDC), women of childbearing age (20-39) in the US had the lowest urine iodine levels of any age group. If you are deficient in iodine, the thyroid just doesn't have the most basic building-blocks to make its key hormones, and all the tissues in the body are negatively impacted as a result.

Selenium

Selenium is another indispensable element in healthy thyroid function. An array of selenium-based proteins and enzymes helps to do several important things. They regulate thyroid hormone synthesis and metabolism; convert T4 into the more accessible form of thyroid hormone, T3; and maintain just the right amount of thyroid hormones in the blood and tissues, including the liver, kidneys and thyroid gland, as well as the brain. Selenium-containing enzymes also function in a protective 'detox' capacity, preserving the integrity of the thyroid gland when we're under all kinds of stress – oxidative, chemical and even social stress. Selenium also helps the body to recycle its iodine stores more efficiently, which can become an important concern as we grow older. Do be aware that, despite its many benefits in the body and the fact that its levels are generally too low in, or even absent from agricultural land, selenium is incredibly toxic in its isolated form. I would never recommend that isolated selenium supplements be used, even though you will find a myriad of them in natural health stores and on the internet. Always get your minerals from food, not pills. The best source of selenium is Brazil nuts.

Zinc, iron and copper

There is no doubt that iodine and selenium are the major players when it comes to trace elements, but there are three trace metals – zinc, iron and copper – that also play vital parts in healthy thyroid function.

Research has shown that both hypothyroidism (underactive thyroid) and hyperthyroidism (overactive thyroid) can sometimes result in a **zinc** deficiency. When zinc levels are low, TSH (thyroid-stimulating hormone), T4 and T3 can in turn become lowered in the body. As for **iron**, research is showing that there is a link between iron deficiency and decreased thyroid function. If you are both anaemic and iodine-deficient, supplementing with iodine alone is unlikely to resolve the thyroid imbalance – you will also need to replenish your iron stores.

Copper is a metal that is needed in trace amounts to produce thyroid-stimulating hormone (TSH). It's also required for T4, so when your body's supply of copper is poor, the rate of T4 production will go down. T4 regulates the body's cholesterol synthesis, and some scientists believe copper deficiency could be what makes people with hypothyroidism more prone to developing high cholesterol and heart problems. Be aware that copper and zinc are in balance with each other. By using an isolated zinc supplement, copper levels are adversely affected, and vice versa for copper reducing zinc levels. Again, isolated supplements are not the answer. The table below indicates the best dietary sources.

Antioxidants and B vitamins

Oxidative stress is what scientists have found to be associated with degenerative diseases and the ageing process in general. You've no doubt heard that antioxidants are good for you. What you often won't hear stated is that there are over 20,000 antioxidants in our food, and we need all of them, not just vitamins A, C, E and selenium.

In hyperthyroidism, the most common form of which is Graves' Disease, oxidative stress can be particularly high. The theory is that because the thyroid is more active, it uses more oxygen, which leads to an accumulation of oxygenated compounds that can harm your cells. This is why antioxidants are recommended, especially in hyperthyroidism.

The B vitamins (B2, B3 and B6) are also important for thyroid function because they are involved in manufacturing T4.

The nutrients I have discussed above can be found in high concentrations in the following foods:

Iodine	*Primary sources*: sea vegetables (kelp, dulse, hijiki, nori, arame, wakame, kombu) *Secondary sources*: asparagus, lima beans, mushrooms, spinach, sesame seeds, summer squash, Swiss chard, garlic
Selenium	Brazil nuts, mushrooms, sunflower seeds (Note: the selenium content of plants is dependent on the selenium levels present in the soil. Much of UK farmland is selenium deficient.)
Zinc	Pumpkin seeds, split peas, whole sprouted grains, sunflower seeds, pecans, Brazil nuts, almonds, walnuts, ginger root
Copper	Shiitake mushrooms, nuts, sprouted chickpeas, sunflower seeds

Iron	Pumpkin seeds, white beans, lentils, spinach, wheatgrass juice
Vitamin A (beta-carotene form)	Kale, sweet potatoes, carrots, winter squash / pumpkin, spinach, cantaloupe melon, broccoli, asparagus
Vitamin C	Guava, kiwi fruit, citrus fruit, strawberries, broccoli, cauliflower, Brussels sprouts, red and orange peppers, camu camu berries, papaya, parsley, greens (kale, turnip, collard, mustard)
Vitamin E	Whole grains, almonds, sprouted beans, sunflower seeds, leafy green vegetables, asparagus
Vitamin B2 (riboflavin)	Brewer's yeast, almonds, wheatgerm, wild rice, mushrooms
Vitamin B3 (niacin)	Brewer's yeast, rice bran
Vitamin B6 (pyroxidine)	Brewer's yeast, sunflower seeds, wheatgerm, sprouted beans, walnuts, brown rice, bananas

A few words about soya consumption

Before we leave the subject of food and thyroid health, it has come to my attention recently that a food that is consistently touted as a health food by many authorities can actually inhibit thyroid function, and therefore is best avoided, no matter what your regular diet is currently. That food is soya (or soy for my American readers).

Soya beans and the products made from them are very far removed from being the health foods that so many companies would have us believe. Let's look at the evidence against the use of soya.

Firstly, approaching 99 per cent of all the soya products on the market are from genetically modified crops. There are two views on the concept of genetic modification. My view is that they are an abomination against nature and will lead to long-term significant adverse consequences that we can't even begin to realise right now in the global experiment that is being conducted on humanity. Strong words perhaps, but this is my personal opinion. Conversely, the multinationals would have us believe that it is the only way we can possibly hope to feed the seven billion people who currently inhabit the planet, and the predicted population of nine billion that is anticipated by 2050. Whatever your personal view, I would not recommend eating genetically modified crops, because we just simply do not know if they will have any long-term health consequences for us; they are relatively new to the scene and therefore insufficient data are available. However, authors and researchers, such as Dr Gabriel Cousens and Dr Brian Clement, are now expressing concern that genetically engineered foods are linked to iodine deficiency and congenital birth defects (Hippocrates Health Institute Magazine *Healing our World*: 33 (4); 14-16).

Secondly, and of importance for those who have not yet made up their minds about the genetic modification issue, we must consider that soya itself, genetically modified or otherwise, has been shown to inhibit thyroid function. If you want thyroid health, soya is off the menu. Soya is also allergenic and for some people quite difficult to digest. Additionally it contains high quantities of phyto-oestrogens, plant chemicals which mimic oestrogen and are being considered now to be detrimental to our sex hormone balance (see above). There is some evidence to suggest that high consumption of soya products, such as those highly processed meat and milk substitutes that are targeted towards vegans, can cause feminisation in men, and even breast cancer in women. This is not a desirable characteristic. We are often told that soya products are good for us, particularly women, because they reduce the incidence of breast cancer. Support for this is extrapolated from the fact that Japanese women regularly consume soya in their traditional diets and have a low incidence of breast cancer. What we are not told, generally, is that it is a different type of soya. Not only is it not genetically modified, it is also fermented, and taken in condiment quantities. This is somewhat different from the blanket extrapolation that would have us believe that these phyto-oestrogens in processed soya products are good for us. Does your diet contain unfermented soya products, such as soya milk, soya cheese, soya meat substitutes, textured vegetable protein and the like? Ask yourself why it is that you feel that you need these non-health-giving foods, and investigate alternatives. You can make your own 'milk' out of almonds, pecans or other nuts. You can make a fabulous 'cheese' from soaked macadamias, cashews and lemon juice with a little crushed garlic. Both taste way better than the processed alternative and will add to, rather than detract from, your health profile.

Gluten

Finally, another thyroid-suppressing 'food' is gluten. As many health-conscious people will be aware, gluten is not actually food. It is a mixture of two insoluble proteins present notably in wheat, and is a substance that gives dough its elasticity. It does not have any nutritional value, but so many processed and otherwise widely accepted foods contain gluten that it can actually be quite hard to avoid it. This sticky protein not only clogs up intestinal functioning and damages the colonic wall, it also inhibits the correct functioning of the thyroid gland. This mechanism seems to be via the reduction of absorption of certain minerals known to be important for thyroid health, notably selenium. Gluten also adversely affects the skin and liver, so going gluten-free is really a no-brainer if our prime objective is optimal health and vitality.

The adrenal glands

The adrenal glands produce two broad types of hormones: adrenocorticoids, our 'stress response' hormones, and mineralocorticoids, those that are responsible for the vital sodium and potassium balance in our bodies – adrenaline and cortisol. We have all heard of the 'fear, fight, flight' response. This is largely due to the production of adrenaline, which prepares us for life-threatening situations in which we have to stand and fight or run for our lives. Amazing things happen to the body during this response, which can produce incredible feats of strength for short periods. We have probably all heard of those stories in which old ladies can lift up cars to release a loved one trapped underneath, much to everyone's amazement, including themselves. This is as a result of the action of adrenaline, which speeds up the heart and respiratory rate, delivers more blood to the muscles, diverts blood away from the digestive system and heightens our awareness of everything. It really can save our life in certain circumstances. The difficulty is that many of us in the modern world experience chronic stress, characterised by both adrenaline and cortisol being secreted regularly in situations which are not in themselves life-threatening. Over time, this leads to many chronic health problems. Since the heart rate is persistently elevated, blood pressure is raised; additionally the digestive system is compromised and the immune system becomes depleted. It has been well documented that sufferers of chronic stress have poor immune function, leading to more frequent illness and a poorer quality of life.

In addition, chronically high cortisol interferes with sleep, and the body's ability to produce other essential hormones, such as DHEA (see page 109), testosterone, oestrogen, progesterone, and thyroid hormone. Over time, excessively high cortisol secretion can contribute to excess abdominal fat, high blood pressure, high blood sugar, and generalised tissue inflammation. In turn, over-production affects DHEA levels, and this in itself compromises bone health, immunity, mood and sex drive.

As the adrenal glands become increasingly depleted, it is more difficult for them to manufacture cortisol. Instead, extra adrenaline is produced to compensate, which can make us irritable and shaky. Adrenal fatigue can cause low blood sugar, anxiety, inability to concentrate, lightheadedness, allergies and low blood pressure. Left unchecked, this points us towards a downward spiral into exhaustion.

According to Dr Sara Gottfried, MD, author of the best-selling book *The Hormone Cure*, when cortisol is in its correct balance, we feel energetic, active and in a good rhythm with life. We don't freak out when under stress, we sleep well and wake feeling restored. We don't crave sugar and our genes can be in 'permanent repair' mode. What a great situation to be in. Cortisol levels can be balanced by changing what we eat, when we eat, and the mood we are in when we eat. This is much better than a commonly pre-scribed medical approach of sleeping pills and anxiety medication.

Rebalancing stress hormones

The following foods absolutely have to be *avoided* to rebalance our stress hormones and rebuild adrenal function:

- Gluten
- Dairy products
- Sugar
- Casein (the protein in milk)
- Processed grains (e.g. white flour)

- Trans-fats (e.g. margarine-type spreads)
- Caffeine.

When timing meals and snacks, it is useful to work with the natural secretion of the adrenal hormones. Cortisol levels naturally start to rise at 6 am, so having a blood sugar-balancing green juice for breakfast is a fantastic way to start the day. If hungry, a second breakfast of, for example, a low glycaemic green smoothie, with some protein powder and maca added, will keep your blood sugar well stabilised until lunch time. Maca, an Andean root, is excellent for adrenal health.

Any adverse stress causes depletion of the adrenal glands, which in turn require organic sodium to replenish them. The best source of organic sodium is celery, which should be part of your daily green juice.

Eating late at night really will disrupt cortisol levels, keeping them abnormally high so that restful sleep is almost impossible. That's why, in addition to it being important for digestive function, I recommend ensuring that nothing is eaten at least three hours before bed time. Overeating at dinner time causes cortisol to spike, and this in turn makes us crave foods that are high in sugar and fat, further disrupting hormone balance. Conversely, according to Dr Gottfried, a glass of water before bed time will lower cortisol levels and make restful sleep more likely.

Alcohol will also play havoc with cortisol levels, due to its sugar content. A couple of glasses of wine to help you relax in the evening is a dangerous habit to get into and helps no one. Love your body enough to avoid doing this to it.

Finally, intense exercise late in the evening causes cortisol levels to remain high. As discussed elsewhere, I certainly do recommend intense exercise, so risking raising your cortisol levels by doing it is not an excuse to stay glued to the sofa. However, it's best to plan your exercise sessions for earlier in the day if you can.

A note about sugar

Sugar consumption in our society is at an all-time high. Could it be that this sweet substance, to which we are so addicted, causes so many health problems? The sugar industry is currently fighting back, trying to convince us, despite massive evidence to the contrary, that sugar is good for us, particularly if we are even remotely athletic. With reference to the adrenal glands, it has been demonstrated that sugar increases our adrenaline production by 400 per cent. We already know how damaging that is, so we absolutely do not want anything to compound our already too high adrenaline levels. Sugar also stresses the pancreas, prevents the central nervous system from functioning correctly, drives minerals out of the body, lowers our immunity and causes dental decay and many other health challenges. These detrimental effects can also be experienced by those eating raw food diets that are excessively high in fruit. To listen to the full story on the dangers of excess sugar consumption, please refer to my CD of the same name, which you can access via my website.

Stress reduction techniques

Stress reduction is essential to fully enjoying one's life experience. Stress-busting techniques include anything from vigorous exercise to meditation to yoga. Everyone is different, so whilst some may let off steam by getting to the gym and bashing a punch bag to within an inch of its life, others may prefer a serene guided visualisation aided by the influence of calming music. Whichever method you choose, ensure that you do it regularly enough to prevent the accumulation of negative stress – something that will slowly but surely undermine the very foundation of your health.

The pituitary gland

The pituitary gland, controlled in turn by the hypothalamus, can be considered to be the master gland of the body. It secretes hormones which are responsible for the regulation of all our other glandular systems, so it is vital that we choose foods that support the pituitary gland in its function. The great news is that the living foods diet is full of all the nutrients that support the production and ultimate functioning of the whole endocrine system. From essential vitamins, minerals, trace elements and fats to oxygen and enzymes, you'll find them all in living food. There's really no need to go into a long individual list. If you're eating your greens, juicing and drinking your sprouts and wheatgrass, eating lots of brightly coloured vegetables every day, and using only whole-food derived, natural supplements, you've got it covered.

The pineal gland

OK, hands up, who's heard of this one? This tiny gland has been referred to as the 'third eye', and it was even proposed by the 17th-century French mathematician and philosopher Rene Descartes to be the seat of the soul. Whilst that cannot be proven scientifically, it seems to have a considerable influence on our mood. The pineal gland produces melatonin, a sleep hormone which is secreted under conditions of dim light. Dim light in the winter months in the higher northern hemisphere can, in many people, lead to a type of depression known as SAD, or seasonal affective disorder. It has been demonstrated that the use of bright light therapy alleviates this condition, and I can personally vouch for its effectiveness, being a SAD person myself. Perhaps the best 'food', therefore, for the pineal gland is bright sunlight. Generally unable to access this in many parts of northern Europe and the USA and Canada for several months of the year, SAD is known to produce signs of mild to moderate depression and even food cravings for processed carbohydrates and sugar. If you find that you have weird food cravings that hit you only in the cold and dark months, it might be the lack of light that is doing it. The best option is, if you can afford it, to take a winter holiday to somewhere hot and sunny. In addition to its mood-boosting effects, it will also allow you to top up your vitamin D levels, which are considered to be too low at the end of summer for many inhabitants above the 50 degrees north line. The alternative is to invest in some full-spectrum lighting bulbs or a 'bright light', which is the next best thing.

Hormones in our food

In addition to the hormone mimickers that have been discussed with particular reference to oestrogen, I can't leave the subject of hormones without considering the effects of the use of growth hormones in animals raised for human consumption. Growth hormones in cattle and sheep have been linked to earlier puberty in girls and the increased risk of breast cancer later in life, as well as the increased incidence of prostate cancer in men. We already know from many studies that the risk of sex hormone-related cancers is higher in meat eaters than in vegetarians. However, vegetarians are not immune, since hormones can also be present in milk. The answer you may be given by the authorities is to eat only organic, hormone-free meat and milk if you are worried. My response is different: I recommend not eating any meat or dairy products at all.

Electromagnetic stress

Electromagnetic stress is a phenomenon that is relatively recent. This 'new kid on the block' is now not only being blamed for its adverse effects on our immune systems, but also the potential derangement of our glandular system in general. Our bodily cells have an electromagnetic frequency, and it is stated by natural health practitioners that this frequency is 75 Hz. Electrical and electronic equipment, particularly the recent insurgence of wireless technology, has the ability to disrupt this delicately balanced frequency and, in turn, has been suggested as a significant cause of deteriorating health. Technology is incredibly useful, and has made our lives infinitely easier, but consider this: it is not many generations ago that we humans were out in nature, farming the land. There was no TV, internet, Facebook or anything of the sort. Adaptable as we are, I don't believe that in the last 70 years we have managed to adapt to this particular assault. I recommend that you wire your computer, minimise your mobile phone usage and turn your phone off at night. Definitely don't leave it next to your bed. It would be easy to say reduce the time you spend in front of a computer, but for most people that's pretty much impossible – after all, we all work with them to some extent. As a method of protecting yourself, look into devices designed to block harmful electromagnetic frequencies (EMFs). Grounding, or 'earthing' yourself, may also be useful, and in the book *Earthing: The Most Important Health Discovery Ever?*, by Clint Ober, Stephen Sinatra and Martin Zucker, the authors recommend earthing devices, or standing barefoot on the grass, as a method of discharging harmful EMFs. It's certainly a technique that I personally use.

A recipe for your hormones: Hijiki-yam medley

This recipe has been kindly contributed by Nomi Shannon, a health educator and living-foods chef from California. Nomi's wonderful book, *The Raw Gourmet* (in which this recipe appears), is a favourite of mine, and highly recommended.

Ingredients

Approx. 30 grams dry weight (1 cup) hijiki (seaweed), soaked (see note)

500 g (2 cups) grated yam

Optional: 4 tablespoons sunflower or pumpkin seeds (if using food combining principles don't use the seeds)

1 tablespoon sesame oil

2 teaspoons grated ginger

2 teaspoons wheat-free tamari

1 pinch cinnamon

- Note: to soak hijiki, place in a small bowl and cover with warm water. Soak for 30 minutes. Drain. Cover again with fresh warm water and let soak another 30 minutes. Drain.
- In a small serving bowl, combine the hijiki, yam, ginger, oil, tamari and cinnamon. Gently toss. Allow flavours to mingle.
- Serves three to four.

Summary

- Oestrogen dominance is a common problem, responsible for many adverse effects
- Several foods have been shown to adversely affect hormonal balance, notably sugar, refined grains, trans-fats, dairy products, soya and anything containing gluten
- In addition to iodine, the thyroid gland requires other essential nutrients for its proper functioning
- The pancreas is easily overworked by high sugar diets
- Fructose consumption, rather than fat consumption, can be more problematic in relation to obesity
- Mood can be elevated by using bright light to stimulate the pineal gland

- We can take in artificial hormones via the food we eat
- Electromagnetic stress is a common issue for everyone working with modern technology.

Chapter 10

The structural system

It takes less effort to smile than to frown.

Our structural elements include the bones, joints, tendons, ligaments, muscles, skin and hair. Numerous foods have been shown to be beneficial for all of these, and still more have been shown to be highly detrimental. Many of the foods that support the other eight systems are also instrumental in the health of our structure, indicating yet again that we can't just compartmentalise our systems. Here, I am going to give a brief overview of bone health, since I have already written a book that details exactly what to do to maintain a strong and healthy skeletal structure well into old age. That book, *Top 10 Raw Food Tips for Osteoporosis*, is available via my website.

Bone health

In women, the age of peak bone density is stated to be at 35; commonly, there is a gradual decline that most women experience after this. I personally do not believe that this gradual decline is natural, but that is what you will read in medical texts. With the right exercise and nutritional considerations, I firmly believe that high bone density can be extended well into old age. Weight training is essential to build bone strength. Without this there can still be a decline, no matter what we eat. The great thing about the living foods regime is that it tends to reduce the bone loss that is promoted by the standard Western diet. Let's take a look at the factors that contribute to bone loss.

- Acidic diet, especially a high-protein diet. This causes increased urinary calcium excretion and draws alkaline mineral reserves out of the body to neutralise the acids from the diet, so that blood pH remains stable between 7.35 and 7.45
- Acidic drinks, such as coffee, fizzy drinks and alcohol
- High salt intake. I do not recommend adding any salt to your recipes
- Smoking. Yet another reason, if anyone needed one, never to smoke
- Lack of weight-bearing exercise. Bone loss is evident within just four days of commencing a sedentary lifestyle
- Pasteurised dairy products. We can't access the calcium in them, no matter what the dairy industry propaganda might try to brainwash us with. They are high fat, high protein and acid forming, so pull minerals from the bones. They also stimulate all stages of the cancer process and should be avoided at all costs
- Lack of sunlight. Vitamin D, formed in the skin on exposure to sunlight, is vital for healthy bone formation. Try to get out in the sun every time it shines. Twenty to 30 minutes is enough. Build up slowly if you are not used to it. There is insufficient sunlight in winter in the UK to build our bones adequately, a good excuse for a winter trip to the tropics, I think.
- Stress, negative thoughts and emotions. These actually have a chemical structure in our bodies and negativity and stress will rot the bones almost as fast as a can of coke. Amazing, isn't it?

Swimming, although excellent for coordination and the cardiovascular system, is non weight-bearing and therefore has no benefit for bone density. A recent study has also indicated that road cycling does not produce a statistically significant increase in bone density.

Muscles, tendons and ligaments

In addition to our bone strength, our muscles, tendons and ligaments are hugely important, and their correct functioning can literally make or break our quality of life. Imagine not being able to run, jump, play and generally fool around as a result of weak or damaged muscles. How many injured sportspeople do we see who might have potentially avoided their injuries with a little more care directed towards their nutrition? A friend of mine who goes to the same gym I attend is a former England cricketer. He now admits he wishes that in his sporting prime he had paid more attention to his diet. The problem is, many young athletes are just that – young, and therefore they believe that they are somehow indestructible. I know I used to.

Athletes are the target for many nutritional products which are of dubious value. I would like, here, to share some information about sports drinks which was originally part of a much longer article that I wrote for my blog.

It has been clearly demonstrated that it is only athletes who have been performing at high intensity for over 90 minutes that might benefit from a drink other than water. However, 'sports drinks' are being marketed to the public in general as performance enhancers. Taking the example of a bright blue drink that I have been offered and declined – called 'berries and tropic fruits', these are fairly typical ingredients:

- Water
- Glucose
- Fructose

- Citric acid
- Mineral salts (sodium chloride, magnesium chloride, calcium chloride, potassium phosphate), flavourings
- Acidity regulator (potassium citrate)
- Stabilisers (acacia gum, glycerol esters of wood rosins)
- Sweeteners (sucralose, acesulfame K)
- Colour (brilliant blue).

Let us review these 'performance enhancing' substances, marketed not only to highly tuned athletes, but also to the mass market, noting that none of them has anything to do with berries or tropical fruits.

Water: OK, unless that water is chlorinated. Unchlorinated, purified water alone would be much better.

Glucose and fructose: These are both sugars. They increase adrenaline production by 400 per cent, stress the pancreas, increase storage of body fat, acidify the body and run minerals out of the bones. They remove enamel from the teeth and feed cancer cells. Listen to my CD, *The Dangers of Excess Sugar Consumption,* for more detail.

Mineral salts: People that sweat do of course need to replace the water-soluble minerals that come out in the sweat, but the listed mineral salts do not adequately do this. They have very limited bioavailability because they are not incorporated into the structure of a plant and have no enzymes attached to them.

Flavourings: I guess these are what enables the manufacturer to call this particular liquid 'berry and tropical fruit blend'. As you can see, there's not a berry, mango or indeed anything else that could be considered to be part of the plant kingdom in the list of ingredients.

Acidity regulator (potassium citrate): In commercial applications, this white crystalline powder is allowed to be contaminated with arsenic and heavy metals (2 ppm [parts per million] and 20 ppm respectively). It is commercially obtained by fermenting glucose syrup (generally from corn) with the aid of the mould *Aspergillus niger* and can be obtained synthetically from acetone (that's nail varnish remover) or glycerol.

Stabilisers (acacia gum, glycerol esters of wood rosins): These additives allow the flavouring oils to mix with the drink and not come out of suspension. The World Health Organisation has recommended that toxicity studies be carried out on these substances, but so far I have not been able to find any.

Sweeteners (sucralose, acesulfame K): Despite glucose and fructose being the primary ingredients after water, it is somehow deemed necessary to add extra sweetness to this concoction. Acesulfame K is 200 times sweeter than sugar and contains the carcinogen methylene chloride, long-term exposure to which can cause headaches, depression, nausea, mental confusion, liver effects, kidney effects, visual disturbances, and cancer in humans. There has been a great deal of opposition to the use of acesulfame K without further testing, but at this time, the FDA has not required that these tests be done. As for sucralose, an artificial sweetener made from sugar, but with more chemical resemblance to the devastating weedkiller DDT than sugar, no long-term toxicity trials have ever been performed. Many users report side effects including gastrointestinal problems, headaches, migraines, blurred vision, allergic reactions and increases in blood sugar levels.

Colour (brilliant blue): Brilliant blue (E133) is a synthetic food dye which has recently been re-evaluated (European Food Safety Authority: EFSA Journal 2010; 8(11):1853), with recommendations to reduce the levels which were previously considered to be acceptable. The EFSA reported no significant carcinogenic activity (although one study cited in this report indicated that at high doses, mutations occurred in rats). Perceived lack of carcinogenicity, however, does not imply that food dyes are therefore harmless. According to an Egyptian study ('Toxic effects of the synthetic food dye Brilliant Blue on liver, kidney and testes functions in rats', Mahmoud, NH. *J. Egypt. Soc. Toxicol,* 2006. Jan:

Vol. 34: 77-84), the author observed that liver enzyme levels in the test animals increased, indicative of liver damage, and that there were abnormalities in the structure of the liver, and congestion and bleeding in the kidneys. Sperm production in the testes of the male animals was also reduced, leading to concerns that, if these animal studies also relate to potential effects on humans, fertility could be adversely affected.

This example is no better or worse than many other sports drinks that are on the market so let me offer some alternatives. Firstly though, judge whether you actually need a performance boost at all by considering which of the following most accurately describes you:

1.   Inactive, does not participate in exercise: Drink water and start exercising.
2.   Participates in exercise for less than 20 minutes per day: Drink water and take more exercise.
3.   Participates in moderate intensity exercise for 20 to 90 minutes per day: Drink water.
4.   Participates in high-intensity exercise for 20 to 90 minutes: Drink water.
5.   Participates in high-intensity exercise for over 90 minutes: Good for you. Drink water. If you feel that your performance level is dropping, drink one of The Raw Food Scientist's special sports drinks which I shall now describe.

You will not find any of my special sports drinks in a shop. You have to make them yourself. There are three different ones.

1.   Green juice. See chapter 1 (page 19).
2.   Coconut water. Get a coconut, drill a hole in the top and drink the liquid contents. Carrying a coconut is difficult, of course, if you are on a long run, bike ride or other discipline, so drink it before you start, or tip the contents

into a (BPA-free) bottle to take round with you.

3.   A mixture of green juice and coconut water.

If you drink any of these, your body will be loaded with antioxidants, you will dilute out the lactic acid produced by the intense exercise and you will feel amazing. In fact, people in all five of the exercise categories I've listed can benefit from green juice and coconut water.

In summary, drinking commercially available sports drinks will not make you a better athlete or miraculously turn you into an athlete. They will, if consumed regularly, shorten and degrade your life. In contrast, drinking my suggested sports drinks will improve your health without supporting companies that profit from people's ignorance.

Sports drinks, energy bars, gel preparations of dubious significance – we may all have seen them. Let's think about what our 'performance' body tissues really need to keep them healthy.

Muscles

Muscles are made of protein. This fact is often sufficient in its own right to spur people who want to grow larger muscles to dash out and grab the latest protein supplement with little concern regarding its true efficacy, or even whether the product they are choosing contains ingredients which could potentially be damaging with long-term use. The main 'ingredient' for muscle growth comes not from what we eat, but from weight training exercise. Humans are actually quite efficient at recycling protein, and the daily quantity of protein we need for all our important functions, including maintenance of the health of our muscles, will generally fit into the palm of the hand.

Researchers from Tufts University studying the effects of protein metabolism during exercise have concluded that adults performing endurance training need 1.5 times the protein intake of sedentary individuals, with those involved in mainly weight and strength training requiring up to twice that of those who do not exercise. Whilst the link between diets high in animal protein and the incidence of cancer and heart disease is well established, research indicates that higher consumption of plant protein does not increase our risk. Recommendations for a balanced spectrum of essential and non-essential amino acids on a raw or high-raw vegan diet include wheatgrass juice, sunflower greens, liquid blue-green algae and hemp, or sprouted brown rice-based protein powders.

Wheatgrass juice is a powerhouse of nutrition which also contains a plethora of elements needed for excellent health. Sunflower greens are an excellent source of complete protein (see page 70), and blue-green algae are over 60 per cent protein. Consuming a green juice containing sunflower sprouts, or a green smoothie which contains protein powder, are both excellent ways of refuelling after strenuous exercise, allowing the muscles to recover and rebuild more quickly.

Muscles require another particularly important nutrient, and that is oxygen. Without oxygen, we would very quickly 'tie up' and be unable to perform. We can see this fact demonstrated particularly well in sprinters. The athlete who wins the 400 metres, the most gruelling of the track sprint distances, is not the one who runs fastest, but the one who slows down the least in the last 100 metres. Muscle is a metabolically active tissue. For its growth and recovery it needs protein, but for recovery, many other factors are essential. During exercise, muscles build up lactic acid. The clue is in the name – the tissue becomes more acidic. So it stands to reason that anything that will reduce the body's overall acidity will enable the muscles to recover faster from their hard work. What gives alkalinity to the body? Green juices, wheatgrass juice, blue-green algae and green leafy vegetables. What detracts from alkalinity? Meat, dairy, processed carbohydrates and grain products, caffeine-containing drinks, sports drinks, cans of fizzy poison... Need I say more? It saddens me greatly still to see so many athletes and 'weekend warriors' delay their opportunity to recover as a result of their misguided food choices. Faster recovery means training can be more frequent, and improvements in speed and strength will be evident faster. Isn't that what we all want?

One of the most aggravating aspects of exercise is feeling stiff and sore afterwards, and sometimes not immediately afterwards – the effect can be noticed anything up to 48 hours after a training session. Whilst building up slowly and not overdoing it are methods of avoiding the pain of DOMS (delayed onset muscle soreness, as this phenomenon is known), this is where nutritional status really can make a difference. Several studies have indicated that DOMS is less severe when vitamin C supplementation is used, whilst others have shown that vitamin C either aggravates the condition or makes no difference. Looking at these studies, I believe they are all flawed to a degree, since they use synthetic vitamin C and not food-source. A synthetic vitamin C supplement will absolutely not do the same thing as a whole-food derived, broad-spectrum supplement that contains all of the approximately 25,000 antioxidants so far discovered, rather than just one of them. A raw or high-raw vegan diet based on green foods and sprouts is an excellent way to boost essential levels of dietary antioxidants. Whole-food supplementation, in my opinion, is also important for anyone who is exercising at high intensity, and is increasingly being used by our Olympians looking for a competitive edge.

As our exercise levels increase, so does the blood flow and oxygen delivery to the muscles. At the same time, energy in the form of ATP is being used up faster than it is being produced. [ATP is our most basic form of energy – it is what our cells need for all their activities.] This, according to research published as long ago as 1990, results in a massive increase in the generation of free radicals (see chapter 4, page 58 for more about free radical damage) via two distinct metabolic pathways. In turn this can exceed the capacity of the cellular defence mechanisms to neutralise them via antioxidant cascades, and lead not only to muscle damage but also potentially to more generalised oxidative damage. The free radical theory of disease is now proven beyond doubt (see chapter 1), and whilst studies using synthetic isolated supplements have been shown to be of no long-term value, whole food supplements containing a broad spectrum of ingredients that provide all the nutrients present in plants are an entirely different proposal, with many recognised benefits. As I recommend to all my clients, and in all my lectures, we need to 'eat the rainbow' – eat as many brightly coloured vegetables as possible to get the broadest spectrum of antioxidant benefits.

Tendons and ligaments

Tendons and ligaments contain similar proteins to the skin. They are easily damaged by not only sports activities but poor eating habits, which detract from their structural integrity. The effects of diets high in foods that are pro-inflammatory will often first be felt in the tendons, ligaments and joints as general stiffness. This is often attributable just to the ageing process, but realistically, there is much that we can do to reverse these ill-effects just by making changes to our meal plans. Standard pro-inflammatory foods are white processed grains, hydrogenated fats, alcohol and any refined foods such as sugar, white bread, pasta and the like. There is a strong correlation between the consumption of white refined sugar and tendon stiffness, giving us yet another reason to ditch the stuff. Anti-inflammatory foods are those which ensure that our metabolic pathways are shifted towards a more beneficial enzymatic cascade (see next section to understand what this means), and include certain essential fatty acids, such as EPA (eicosapentaenoic acid – see below).

All fives and sixes?

The enzymatic cascades that are responsible for the conversion of linoleic acid to gamma linolenic acid, ultimately giving us either pro-inflammatory or anti-inflammatory prostaglandins (a type of hormone), are the delta 5 and delta 6 desaturases. In a nutshell, the more delta 5 we have, the more we convert to pro-inflammatory prostaglandins. The more delta 6 we have, the more anti-inflammatory effect we can create. Delta 6 desaturase is inhibited by trans-fats, sugar, stress and alcohol, leading us into inflammatory decline and accelerated ageing, which I guess not many of us would voluntarily vote for. Delta 5 desaturase activity is increased by elevated insulin levels, which helps to explain why type 2 diabetes and dietary practices which spike our insulin levels send us on the path to poor health via creating inflammatory processes in the body. The activity of the bad guy, delta 5 desaturase, can be reduced via an increased intake of EPA. Read many health articles and you will begin to believe that the only source of EPA is fish oil, which personally I do not recommend; I suggest reading *Killer Fish*, by Brian Clement, for further information on the damaging aspects of fish oil. The fish, however, obtain their EPA from algae, and seaweed also contains EPA. As I state in chapter 5, I therefore recommend that you 'eat like a fish' for your EPA and consider freshwater algae as a good source of this important anti-inflammatory fat.

Skin

The largest and most visible of our organ systems, the skin is a true reflection of our health and the first thing that people see. Glowing skin is easy to achieve on a living foods regime, and there are many ways in which a healthy diet supports it. From the incessant advertising of skin creams and serums, we could be forgiven to believe that we could eat anything we liked and, as long as we use the latest serum costing upwards of $200 per bottle, all will be well. Sorry – you're going to be disappointed. I certainly believe that the best way to improve your skin is by eating well.

Staying on the subject of facial creams for just a moment, I would always recommend that before you put anything on your face, or anywhere else on your body for that matter, you check the list of ingredients. If you wouldn't eat it, don't put it on your skin, because you are going to absorb it. Ever wondered why the skin patch is such an effective means of delivering everything from hormones to painkillers? Stuff goes in... It is genuinely frightening when you read about the concoctions of harsh, aggressive chemicals that people use as 'anti-ageing', 'contouring' (whatever that means!), 'rejuvenating', and, laughably, 'age-defying' cosmetics. It almost seems that the longer the list of unpronounceable chemicals, the more the company can charge for their product. I picked up an expensive eye cream whilst at a very smart spa in December 2012, and wrote down the list of ingredients. This *Revitalising Eye Contour Cream*, manufactured in France, and stated to be for professional use only, is supposed to be 'firming' and bring a youthful look to the eye area and banish wrinkles. I hasten to add that I put it straight back on the shelf after writing down the long list of chemical constituents present. Here it is:

Water, Cetearyl alcohol, Liquid paraffin, Propylene glycol, Stearic acid, Beeswax, Lanolin, Alcohol, Sodium cetearyl sulphate, Sodium lauryl sulphate, Triethanolamine, Phenoxyethanol, Perfume, Cyclopentasiloxane, Hazel leaf extract, Hyssopus officinalis *extract,* Anthemis nobilis *flower oil, Hydrolysed elastin, Benzoic acid, Dimethiconol, Dehydroacetic acid, Ethylhexylglycerin, Methylparaben, Butylparaben, Ethylparaben, Isobutylparaben, Propylparaben, Citronellol, Linalool, Hydroxycitronellal, Hexyl cinnamal, Limonene, Geraniol, Coumarin, Alpha-isomethyl ionone, Hydroxyisohexyl 3-cyclohexine, Carboxaldehyde.*

Amongst the chemical ingredients in this list, we have six potential carcinogens – the five 'parabens'– according to one toxicology study (Daubre PD, Aljarrah A, Miller WR, Coldham NG, Sauer MJ, Pope GS, 'Concentrations of parabens in human breast tumours', *Journal of Applied Toxicology* 2004; 24: 5-13), and phenoxyethanol (Carvalho CM, Menezes PF, Letenski GC, Praes CE, Feferman IH, Lorencini M, 'In vitro induction of apoptosis, necrosis and genotoxicity by cosmetic preservatives: application of flow cytometry as a complementary analysis by NRU', *International Journal of Cosmetic Science* 2012; 34(2): 176-182), several potential allergens (the parabens, phenoxyethanol and ethylhexylglycerin), neurotoxic agents (again, the parabens) and, in my opinion, absolutely nothing that would be likely to improve the appearance of the skin in any part of the body. Compare this with the list of somewhat more pronounceable ingredients present in the facial moisturiser that I use (made by a UK company called Raw Gaia):

Cold pressed cacao butter, Cold pressed oils of apricot kernel, Evening primrose, Rosehip, Essential oils of palmarosa, rose geranium, lavender.

No chemicals, no carcinogens, no toxic sunblock, nothing questionable, nothing synthetic. The product is packaged in dark glass to prevent degradation and rancidity of the oils and it has a recommended shelf life of six months, again so that there is no chance of spreading rancid oil onto the skin. What a difference.

I also have a total aversion to sunblock, and only recommend its use if you are very pale and are visiting the tropics or are climbing a mountain. The ridiculous suggestion that we need factor 50 on the body before we even venture outside is a known contributor to the rapidly escalating occurrence of rickets in the UK, with orthopaedic surgeons at the University of Southampton reporting that they are seeing up to 20 new cases per day. We are so paranoid of skin cancer that we spread toxic chemicals all over ourselves without so much as a thought. Here's the thing – we need sun exposure. It boosts the immune system. It aids in detoxification. It elevates our mood and increases our vitamin D levels, vital for bone health and cancer prevention. People with low vitamin D levels as a result of inadequate sun exposure risk serious health problems. The best sunblock is loose fitting cotton clothes, and if you have to use something on exposed skin, then a product called Caribbean Blue, available via the Fresh Network in the UK, is a non-toxic sunblock that I use on my face when I am up mountains. Take a look at the ingredients in your sunblock today. Is it time for a change of product, or your perceived relationship with the sun?

The first point to consider when aiming for healthy looking skin is hydration. We spoke all about this in chapter 8 in regard to the kidneys, which are our water regulation system. We want to remain hydrated otherwise our skin will be one of the first things to suffer. Funnily enough, I recommend drinking green juice every day for beautiful skin. I wonder, where might you have read about green juice before?

Food for the skin

When thinking about food that enhances our skin, we're thinking of food that not only improves our water balance and hydration, but also incorporates the structural elements we need to renew our skin cells. Let's have a look at some skin food now.

Grapefruit and blueberries

Both grapefruit and blueberries contain good levels of vitamin C, which is essential in the synthesis of collagen. If the skin lacks collagen, it is more prone to wrinkling and appears older. Blueberries are also high in lycopene, as are tomatoes, which is a nutrient that has been found to give us some protection against sun damage. Watermelon is also a good source of lycopene, and, with a water content of 92 per cent, it is a great hydrator.

Spinach and other dark greens

Yet again here are the green foods coming to our rescue, this time for vanity's sake! The dark green leafy vegetables are known to contain compounds which have the ability to reverse damage to cellular DNA in the skin. Yet another good reason to add spinach, kale, cavolo nero and other dark green leaves to your morning juice.

Almonds

Almonds, particularly if soaked and sprouted, are fantastic for skin due to their vitamin E content. Avocados are likewise beneficial for the same reason.

Food supplements

A recent study conducted in 2012 indicated that Juice Plus fruit and vegetable capsules, which I have previously mentioned, had benefits for skin as a result of improving its thickness and positively affecting the skin's microcirculation. Experts at the skin research centre at the University of Witten/Herdecke in Germany saw improvements in skin density, thickness and hydration in 52 women over a 12-week period.

MSM (methyl sulphonyl methane)

MSM is an interesting supplement which provides a form of organic sulphur (see below). Remember from chapter 9 (page 111) that MSM also acts as a methyl donor and is therefore useful for the detoxification of bad oestrogen. Naturally occurring MSM is easily destroyed by food processing and constant utilisation and excretion by the body; supplementation may be necessary to meet bodily requirements.

MSM is a white, crystalline, water-soluble, odourless and almost tasteless powder. It is neither a drug or food additive but what could be termed 'a nutritional mineral'. Even moderate processing can drive it out of our food, making its benefits unavailable to us. Commercially, it is made either via distillation or crystallisation, with distillation generally regarded as producing a purer product.

The list of sulphur uses in the body is extensive. It is essential for the development of hair, nails and skin, connective tissue and enzymes, hormones and immunoglobulins. Experimental findings suggest that MSM has a biological role as a cell wall stabilising factor.

MSM was considered to be an important factor in the diets of our ancestors as far back as the middle ages. It is found in plants which are grown using the cycles of rain, and absent from plants grown in modern-day greenhouses or those dependent on watering via irrigation. Since most modern-day diets in developed countries include an alarming quantity of processed food, MSM is now likely to be present only in very small quantities, or completely absent.

The chief benefits of MSM are:

Hair, skin and nails: Sulphur is necessary for the production of collagen and keratin. These proteins are essential for the health and maintenance of hair, skin and nails. Collagen binds the structures of skin together while keratin is the primary component in hair, nails, skin and tooth enamel. MSM enhances tissue pliability and encourages repair of damaged skin.

Bones, joints and ligaments: Sulphur is critical in the formation of collagen and glucosamine, which are vital components of healthy bones, joints, ligaments and tendons. Sulphur also makes cells more permeable, allowing nutrients and fluids to flow freely through the cells and remove toxins, ultimately reducing pain and inflammation.

Allergies: MSM is said to help fortify the body's natural barriers against allergens.

Respiratory system: MSM helps strengthen the lungs, possibly regulating the fluid that covers the surface of the airways.

Carbohydrate metabolism: Sulphur is needed to produce insulin and other vital components that contribute to healthy carbohydrate metabolism. MSM helps make the cells more permeable allowing them to absorb blood sugar. Alpha lipoic acid, a sulphur-containing compound, plays a part in the generation of energy and in glucose balance.

Gastrointestinal system: MSM helps promote good digestive function and absorption of nutrients.

Sulphur-containing foods

Most of the sulphur found in the body is incorporated into keratin, which gives substance to the skin, nails and hair. Sulphur must be present for the body to produce collagen, which keeps skin soft and supple. That's why sulphur is often referred to as the beauty mineral. Sulphur is found in every cell in the body. It is structurally and functionally important to 150 compounds, including tissues, enzymes, hormones, antibodies and antioxidants. Organic sulphur is known for its anti-inflammatory and circulation-enhancing properties.

Sulphur is present in many of the foods that we eat. The best plant sources are garlic, onions, Brussels sprouts, kale, wheat germ and asparagus. We can also boost our intake of sulphur by using MSM, as mentioned above.

Sulphur has a long history for use as a health and beauty mineral. The ancient Romans soaked themselves in sulphuric waters to relieve pain and to prevent ageing.

Dry skin brushing and lymphatic drainage massage will also have benefits for the appearance of the skin.

Joints

Joint health is a huge subject to consider, and a book in its own right (in fact, the book I'm writing next will be on the subject of joint health). According to the charity Arthritis Care, there are approximately 10 million people in the UK alone who have arthritis, and the impact this has on their lives, and the subsequent burden of care this places on the National Health Service, is massive. For this joint health section, I am not going to write my next book and insert it here. What I will do is list the things that we know are detrimental to joint function, and then follow up with those things that we know to be beneficial, and can restore our mobility and function.

Factors that detract from healthy joints

Obesity

In addition to the extra strain put on the joints by carrying excessive weight, it has now been shown that high levels of adipose (fatty) tissue produce their own pro-inflammatory chemicals which aggravate the joints. Obese people often state that they cannot exercise, especially if they have joint pain. However, by exercising in water, which everyone can do, even obese people with painful joints can benefit not only from exercise which helps with joint mobility, but also from burning off excess caloric intake which led to the obesity in the first place. Diet, however, has to be improved as well, since exercise alone will not supply the nutrients needed for the creation of healthier new cells.

High-sugar diets

As discussed elsewhere, high sugar consumption creates tissue damage which can affect every part of the body, not just the joints. It also tips the body towards inflammation and increases levels of inflammatory cytokines. Kicking the sugar habit can be hard – it does, after all, act like an addictive drug. However, it is absolutely essential to eliminate the harmful sugar that is well known to degrade the cells prematurely.

Meat and dairy product consumption

The excess protein in these foods can tip the body towards the process of 'glycation', as previously described (chapter 9, page 117), which in turn leads to the generation of free radicals. Free-radical damage to the joints precipitates the development of arthritis. Excess protein from animal sources is also well known to aggravate gout, the painful accumulation of uric acid crystals in the joints. Alcohol also makes gout worse, as well as being directly damaging to the joints (see below).

Adverse omega-3 to omega-6 fatty acid ratios

Most people have this challenge. The ideal ratio of omega-3 to omega-6 fatty acids should be 2:1, but due to the chronic consumption of trans-fats from hydrogenation, the processing of fats until they no longer resemble the plant they came from, and frying food in rancid vegetable oil, we generally have a ratio that is far removed from the ideal, with way too much omega 6. Supplementation with omega-3 fats has been shown to relieve joint pain and improve mobility, but beware, again, of the fish-oil salesmen. The best plant sources of omega-3 fats are blue-green algae, chia seed and hemp oil.

Alcohol

You will still hear that wine is good for the heart, no matter what we know about how it wrecks the liver and kills brain cells. Alcohol is particularly bad for your joints too, due to its sugar content and the fact that it causes increased tissue acidity.

Oxidative stress

Free radicals damage the synovial membrane of the joints as well as the articular cartilage. We need a high intake of dietary antioxidants from eating a rainbow plant-based diet. Whole food supplementation will also reduce free-radical damage.

Smoking
This ghastly habit creates massive numbers of free radicals which destroy our health, prematurely age us and send us to an early grave. There is no safe limit for tobacco usage.

Pro-inflammatory lifestyle choices
Basically, all the things that we currently know are bad for us – smoking, alcohol, processed meat, dairy products, fast food, fizzy drinks, inactivity. All will lead to a rapid demise of joint mobility and function.

Lack of exercise
Whilst there will be people who insist that excessive exercise degrades the joints, such as, for example, long-distance running, a lack of exercise can be just as damaging for us. Weak muscles can lead to poor posture, which itself can lead to joint aggravation and dysfunction, and failing to move a joint through its full range of motion can reduce oxygenation and decrease detoxification.

Beneficial nutrients for joints

Kelp
High in fibre, this brown seaweed reduces inflammation, is high in antioxidants and has anti-cancer properties. All seaweed is wild food which contains all eight of the essential sugars (glucose, galactose, xylose, fucose, mannose, N-acetyl glucosamine, N-acetyl galactosamine, N-acetyl nicotinic acid). Deficiency in any of the essential sugars can lead to neurological problems as well as problems with joints and connective tissue. These essential sugars are also found in mushrooms and edible flowers.

Extra virgin olive oil
The secret to longevity in Mediterranean culture, this oil provides mono-unsaturated fats that fight inflammation, can help

lower risks of asthma and arthritis, as well as protect the heart and blood vessels. Olive oil is also a natural aromatase inhibitor, as is passionflower. Aromatase, also known as 'oestrogen synthase', is an enzyme involved in one of the stages in the production of oestrogen. Aromatisation (chemical alteration involving the enzyme aromatase) of androgenic (male) hormones, notably testosterone, leads to an increase in bad oestrogen (see chapter 9), so any food that naturally puts the brakes on this conversion – that is, the aromatase inhibitors – will be beneficial in the fight against oestrogen dominance and its detrimental effects.

Cruciferous vegetables
Broccoli, Brussels sprouts, kale and cauliflower are all loaded with antioxidants. Naturally detoxifying and anti-inflammatory, they can help rid the body of harmful compounds.

Blueberries
Blueberries not only reduce inflammation, but also protect the brain from ageing and prevent diseases such as cancer and dementia. Aim for organic berries, since berries in general are one of the most highly sprayed crops.

Turmeric
This powerful yellow spice contains curcumin, a natural anti-inflammatory compound. It is said to have an equivalent effect to non-steroidal anti-inflammatory drugs, but without their adverse side effects. Turmeric is also a spice which is highly prized for its anti-cancer benefits.

Ginger
In addition to its benefits for the circulatory system, ginger helps to reduce inflammation and control blood sugar. Why not add some to your green juice every day?

Garlic

As well as its benefits for the immune system and circulation, garlic can help to reduce inflammation.

Sweet potato

A great source of complex carbohydrates, fibre, beta-carotene, manganese and vitamins B6 and C, these potatoes actually help heal inflammation in the body. Try them grated on salads or in a juice.

White potato juice

Juiced white potatoes are a fantastic treatment for arthritis and raw potato juice is widely used in Scandinavian clinics as an arthritis treatment. It is interesting to note that as a member of the nightshade family, white potatoes only have their benefits when used raw. Cooked white potatoes are pro-inflammatory and actually cause damage to the joints. To take white potato juice, run the potatoes through the juicer and leave the juice until the starch settles to the bottom of the glass before drinking.

Some misconceptions about joint health

Prior to leaving a discussion on joint health, ensure that you avoid the things that we may in the past have been told are good for joints. Firstly, **cod liver oil**. This is dreadful stuff. It is extracted from the liver of a large fish, close to the top of the food chain, which is contaminated with mercury and organophosphates, to name but two harmful compounds. It is very high in vitamin A, which in turn inhibits the action of osteoblasts, our bone-building cells. It is no coincidence that the countries with the highest cod liver oil consumption also have the highest incidence of osteoporosis.

Secondly, despite massive promotion of **glucosamine** and **chondroitin** as health supplements for joints, a recent study questioned their use and found that they made negligible difference to joint health and mobility. Remember that degenerative joint disease (arthritis) is a dynamic process which holds a balance between degeneration and regeneration. It used to be thought that once arthritis began, the only way was towards degeneration, but this is now known to be untrue. We can influence whether the balance is tipped in favour of further degeneration, or regeneration, purely via our food and lifestyle choices. A healthy living foods-based diet that minimises fruit (sugar) consumption is the best choice for regeneration. Incorporating exercise every day, in water if necessary to relieve joint stress, will allow you to repair and recover from this debilitating condition.

Hair

Hair is indeed part of our structure, and shiny, lustrous hair is a sure sign of good health. Isn't it amazing that, when people see someone with lovely hair, they often ask them which shampoo they use? Shampoo generally has little or nothing to do with hair health – it once again comes down to what we are eating that dictates how good our hair looks. My top two tips for great hair are as follows – seaweed and sulphur. I was amazed at how fast my hair grew when I first started eating seaweed regularly. Everything that is good for the skin, as mentioned above, will be good for the hair. Avoid using harsh chemicals on the hair, don't wash it too frequently and don't dye it! Many hair dyes use known carcinogens and are absorbed through the scalp. Check your shampoo for the presence of sodium laureth (lauryl) sulphate (SLS) and parabens. SLS is used in industrial floor-cleaning applications, and you don't want that on your hair. Parabens are potentially carcinogenic (see page 146). Anything that you wash your hair in can be absorbed through the scalp, so look at your shampoo in the same way as you would a face cream – would it be safe to consume it?

Grey hair?

A common concern as we age is the appearance of grey hair. It is often viewed as a sign that our youth is finally over. Greying of the hair is caused by depigmentation of the shaft, which in turn often correlates to a mineral deficiency, notably that of copper and zinc. This is not the time to go rushing out and buying a copper or zinc supplement, however. As I stated previously, if you supplement with copper, you reduce your zinc levels, and vice versa. The best sources of minerals for the reversal of greying hair are wheatgrass juice and seaweed. Wheatgrass has the capacity to take up to 92 minerals out of the soil and incorporate it into its structure. By growing your own wheatgrass, especially if you enrich the soil it is grown in, you can feed your body not just with the minerals needed for natural hair colour, but up to 90 others which have massive benefits for each system. I use a liquid fertiliser called Ocean Solution, which is diluted ocean water, to feed my wheatgrass. There are many established benefits of using diluted ocean water for growing your own food, and the best book to read on this subject is *Sea Energy Agriculture*, by Maynard Murray. You can also use rock dust mixed in with the soil to get your wheatgrass to take up more minerals.

Have you ever experienced a head massage? Massaging the scalp will increase the blood flow to this area, which in turn has benefits for the hair follicles and therefore the hair itself. Whilst you can perform your own scalp massage, having an Indian head massage, a technique practised in India for over 1000 years but only introduced to the West in 1970, brings a wonderful sense of relaxation and well-being. Not only is the head massaged, but the upper back, neck and face are also treated. These are the areas in which we hold most of our tension, so an Indian head massage brings relaxation, which in turn has benefits for the nervous system, immune system, structural system, lymphatic system and respiratory system.

A recipe for good structure: Kelp noodles with shiitake-kale pesto

This recipe was kindly contributed by Jessica Li, a raw food chef and personal trainer from Canada. It is ideal for structural bone health. Kale is high in calcium and the vitamin D found in shiitake mushrooms aids the body's absorption of calcium.

Ingredients

6 oz/150 grams kelp noodles

2 handfuls (1 cup) basil

3 handfuls (1 ½) cups green kale

60 g (¼) cup pine nuts

3-4 tablespoons cold pressed extra-virgin olive oil

½ teaspoon sea salt

1 clove garlic, crushed

3 teaspoons lemon juice

¼ cup of dried shiitake mushrooms (soak in water until soft)

¼ cup spinach

¼ water

- Soak the 6 oz of kelp noodles (about half a small package) in warm water and a tablespoon of lemon juice, or apple/cider vinegar, for at least 30 minutes to soften noodles. Rinse noodles well and set aside.
- Process everything in a food processor until well blended and smooth. Toss with kelp noodles. Garnish with sprigs of parsley (optional).

Summary

- Osteoporosis is a silent epidemic. Weight-bearing exercise, correct hormonal balance, sun exposure and stress reduction are all essential for maintaining bone health

- Muscle growth is more dependent upon weight training than protein intake, although active people do need more protein than sedentary individuals; this is best obtained from plant sources
- Tendons and ligaments require an anti-inflammatory lifestyle for their health
- Skin absorbs all the substances that you put on it. You can add to, or detract from, the health of your skin by what you eat, as well as by using cosmetics
- Joints are massively affected by diet and lifestyle. Obesity and lack of exercise are very damaging to the joints, as are alcohol and sugar consumption
- Grey hair can be an indication of mineral deficiency. This can often be reversed by using highly mineral-dense plant foods such as wheatgrass juice, combined with an excellent diet.

Chapter 11

General recommendations

...To enhance all of your systems!

This is one of those chapters that could go on and on, and take on a life of its own. I therefore felt that I should systematise this summary, mainly to prevent this book becoming a 500-page tome of 'everything you always wanted to know about healthy food and lifestyles but were afraid to ask...'. In this section, I'll cover the sort of things that will make your day go even better. If we pay attention not just to what we eat, but when we eat it, and how we eat it, then we can squeeze even more juice out of life.

First, I recommend to all my clients that they should gradually increase the proportion of sprouted food that they eat. This needs to be a gradual process since it takes time for the gut microflora to adapt to the change, and you don't want to be producing a lot of gas. Following 50 years of study with guests at the Hippocrates Health Institute, it has been indicated that the ideal level is to have 20 to 25 per cent of the diet as sprouted food for optimal health and vitality. Below is a list of the six categories of sprouted foods:

Large greens, grown in soil: These include wheatgrass, sunflower greens, pea shoots and buckwheat. Their chlorophyll content is very high, and they are excellent sources of magnesium and many other essential minerals. Ideally it's great to grow these foods yourself, but you can also order them in from companies that will deliver them to your home, depending on where that is. No green juice is complete without them.

Small green leafed sprouts: These are grown without soil, in jars or in an automatic sprouter. They include alfalfa, broccoli, clover and radish, and have remarkable health benefits, particularly in relation to the prevention of cancer. They are classified as a vegetable – make sure that all your salads contain some of these little powerhouses of nutrition.

Grain sprouts: These include wheat, barley, quinoa, amaranth. They are carbohydrate dominant, so don't combine them with proteins. They are easily grown in a jar.

Carbohydrate sprouts: These include lentils and chickpeas. Don't combine with proteins. They are also easily grown in jars.

Neutral sprouts: These can be mixed with everything. Mung and aduki are the only ones in this category. They are grown in jars, in the same way as grain and carbohydrate sprouts.

Fenugreek sprouts: These are in a category of their own. They have a gentle energy and are great for stabilising blood sugar and eliminating body odour. They are spicy. Grow them in a jar, or in an automatic sprouter if you want to grow them on to produce a green-leafed sprout.

I recommend eating sprouted food because the nutritional content is so high, and it is in a form which is more easily digested. Some authors even refer to sprouted food as being 'pre-digested'. Sprouts are second only to seaweeds for mineral content, and they can even rival the seaweeds if they are grown in highly mineralised soil.

I have included a recipe at the end of each chapter, but one thing that I was adamant about was that this book was not going to become a recipe book. I'll let you into a secret – I'm pretty hopeless at creating recipes. It goes without saying that I love my healthy food and my whole lifestyle, but one of the things that I really don't have time to do is spend hours in the kitchen. Most of my meals are thrown together in just five to 10 minutes, and if you came to dinner it wouldn't be particularly elaborate. To make up for my shortcomings, in the resources section you will find a list of some excellent recipe books which support the recommendations that I have made in the preceding chapters.

Below I have listed some meal suggestions for a typical day following the lifestyle that I recommend, which supports the whole body. Remember to get some exercise in as well.

Breakfast

I recommend that most people keep breakfast very light, unless the individual has difficulty in maintaining body weight. This serves to extend the period of detoxification from the last meal the previous day. Here I have broken breakfast down into five stages. Not everyone has the luxury of five breakfasts – indeed, critics would argue that no one has time for such indulgence. However, once people get into a routine with this, it doesn't take a lot of time and could even take less time overall than stopping off at the coffee shop on the way to work.

1. On rising, a glass of pure water with freshly squeezed lemon juice and a pinch of cayenne pepper. The water can be warm, hot or cold, but body temperature is best. The reason is that it takes energy to cool liquids down to body temperature, and it also takes energy to warm them up if iced. Since a challenge for so many people

is a lack of energy, we don't want to waste any. This combination is alkalising and hydrating, and improves both circulation and digestive strength.

2.   For those who are using it, wheatgrass juice next, after about 10-15 minutes. Wheatgrass juice is nature's perfect medicine. It is highly mineralised, draws heavy metals out of the body, aids in detoxification, boosts the immune system, alkalises, improves tissue oxygenation by boosting haemoglobin formation in the blood... it is wondrous stuff, and it tastes *great*. If it makes you feel a bit nauseous, try having a bit less. Two fluid ounces in the morning is really all you need, although if you're feeling brave you could take it twice daily. Swill it around in your mouth a bit before swallowing. If two fluid ounces is too much, do one ounce initially and gradually increase over a few days.

3.   Deep breathing in the garden (if you are lucky enough to have one) for five to 10 minutes. If you feel a bit light-headed initially, it's because of CO_2 'washout'; have a rest for two minutes then start again. This can be considered to be a breakfast, since you are feeding your cells with oxygen. As part of your daily routine you'll see improvements in your respiratory system in no time. Instead of this breakfast, some people may choose exercise at this time, which as we know boosts the mood, the respiratory and cardiovascular systems and helps with our structural strength. Alternatively, some may choose to meditate at this time of day. This feeds the mind, so counts as a breakfast too.

4.   The most important part of the day (about 15 minutes after wheatgrass) – green juice time. The daily green juice is an absolute staple of the recommended Hippocrates lifestyle and you need a good juicer for this. Green juices alkalise, remineralise, rehydrate, feed and oxygenate the

cells and charge up the immune system. They should be compulsory in schools and hospitals. My green juice recipe is given in chapter 2 (page 19). Throw everything through the juicer in no particular order (for some reason I put the sprouts through first, then the celery and cucumber, but this is not important), and drink within five minutes of making it. Swill it around in your mouth first before swallowing. This starts the digestive process. You can make up extra juice and keep it in the fridge until it's time to make an evening soup if you like. You will lose some of the enzymes by doing this, but many of the other beneficial nutrients will be preserved. Add ginger for warmth, lime for tang and kale for extra protein and minerals if you fancy it. And don't forget the garlic for the immune system.

5.   Finally, if you are still hungry, half an hour after green juice, ripe tomatoes make an excellent breakfast for those with blood sugar or fungal issues who are avoiding fruit. They have a low glycaemic index (as discussed previously, an indication of how rapidly, or otherwise, sugar is absorbed into the blood stream from food; generally, the lower the better), easily digested, alkalising (see page 20) and liver-cleansing. If you are using tomatoes as a breakfast, avoid eating anything else until two hours later, in case you have problems with food combining. Tomatoes take two hours to digest. Other options if not having tomatoes include sprouted buckwheat cereal, either dehydrated or not, with almond or quinoa milk, or some blueberries, which have a low glycaemic index, but you may prefer to avoid them altogether if they affect your blood sugar balance.

As an alternative, for 'fifth breakfast', I now use a fantastic breakfast made of chia seed. Chia seed is the latest superfood to hit the news in nutritional science and it really is wonderful stuff (see the recipe at the end of chapter 3). Put a couple of dessert-spoons of the seed in a bowl, add home-made or shop-bought almond milk (home-made is far better), wait 15 to 20 minutes, stirring occasionally. This gives a porridge-style breakfast that is very high in omega-3s, an excellent protein source and also a fantastic source of fibre. I challenge anyone to be constipated on chia porridge.

Snacks

Here are two very easy options to keep you going:

Soaked seeds or nuts: Almonds are the most easily digestible. Remove the skins before eating. Soaking removes the enzyme inhibitors, which is very important. Any seeds can be used. If you prefer a crunchy texture, seeds can be soaked overnight, then dried in the dehydrator. This is not mad, since we soak seeds to get rid of enzyme inhibitors. I always feel better eating nuts and seeds that have not been re-dried, because they contain organic water and are therefore easier on the digestive system. When using nuts and seeds as a snack, remember the food-combining rule – no carbohydrate-dominant foods within four hours to optimise digestive function. Always chew nuts and seeds thoroughly.

Crackers: Home made in a dehydrator for those who care to follow one of the recipes in the books I recommend, or raw shop-bought, these make a great snack and can be incorporated into lunch. Most crackers will be grain based so remember to check ingredients with respect to food combining. Sprouted grain-based crackers are a great source of fibre and combine well with home-made hummus. A quick hummus recipe would be sprouted chickpeas, lemon juice, garlic and a pinch of spice. Use the juicer with the blank screen (see page 193) to process the chickpeas; then add crushed garlic, lemon juice and spices afterwards. Very easy! Chickpeas sprout well in a jar.

Lunch

I always recommend a large green salad as the base for any lunch. If you are eating your proteins at lunch time, greens combine well with these. Your proteins can either be mixed in with the salad or present in the sauce, for example a seed-based sauce is quite popular. This is where you can really get going with your sprouted foods, which are easily digestible and give you energy. I generally throw some or all of the following into my salads: rocket, watercress, spinach, kale, dandelion, lamb's lettuce, coriander (good for getting rid of heavy metals), parsley, mizuna, seaweed... basically anything dark green. To this I will add any of the following sprouts – radish, sunflower, broccoli, alfalfa, mung, onion, clover. Then I add a load of chopped vegetables, such as radish, peppers (excluding green peppers as they are not ripe) and anything brightly coloured, and maybe some avocado, lemon juice and raw vegan pesto (I cheat and buy this in a jar). If you are increasing your garlic consumption, for either immunity or circulation, or both, add one to two cloves of crushed garlic with your salad. I don't like to mix too many fats at lunch, so if I am using avocado in the salad I will avoid a seed dressing.

If this type of living foods diet is new to you and you feel you are detoxing too quickly, have some steamed vegetables for lunch. These combine well with steamed grains such as amaranth or quinoa (best to sprout them first), or a baked sweet potato or baked squash. This is also good if you are craving cooked food or feeling the psychological need for warmth. Raw ways of feeling warmer are to add chillies or ginger to your salads or sauces, and consider adding a one-inch slice of ginger to your juices. Ginger can also be used grated into soups.

Dinner

If you enjoy playing around with food, I can recommend any of the recipes from the Hippocrates book as dinner choices. I also like the idea of blended food in the late afternoon or evening since it is easier to digest. Why not try the soup recipe at the end of chapter 2? Soups are excellent because you can throw in pretty much anything that's a vegetable and the blender will forgive you. It may turn out to be a slightly odd colour, as many of my soups do, but if you're not trying to impress anyone else with them it really doesn't matter. Soups can be used warm as well, either by warming them up in a dehydrator, or putting the bowl of soup into a bowl of hot water, stirring regularly, for 10 to 15 minutes. I suggest that if you are using the carbohydrate-dominant foods, such as the small alkalising grains or the legume sprouts, you have them at dinner time.

Ensure you eat your last meal at least three hours before going to bed if you can. I recommend this because the sleeping hours are then used for what they are intended for – assimilation, detoxification, recovery and rebuilding.

Timing of drinking is also important. Avoid drinking within half an hour before, or two hours after, your meals. This is to ensure that you do not dilute your digestive enzymes. We're all so used to drinking with our meals that it might seem a little odd to those unfamiliar with this way of eating to avoid water at this time. However, that is the recommendation; try it and see how your digestion improves.

Basic food recommendations

These are the guiding principles behind this book:

Eat organic: It is best to eat only organic produce. Many studies have shown that the nutritional value of organic food is higher than that of conventionally grown food. It also is free from environmental toxins (see below) and supports a more natural approach to farming.

Raw is best: Try to eat as much uncooked food as possible. Ideally, cooked food should be kept to just 20 per cent of the diet by weight. The healthiest cooked choices are steamed vegetables, baked squashes and sweet potatoes and lightly cooked alkalising grains such as quinoa, amaranth, teff, buckwheat and millet. Limit fruit consumption to one to two pieces per day and focus on the green foods and fresh vegetables in abundance. Soak and sprout all seeds, grains and legumes before eating them, whether you are cooking them or not. Eliminate processed grains and dairy products since they are acid-forming and tend to aggravate mucus production.

Avoid meat and animal products: As I have said many times throughout this book, I do not recommend eating meat. Despite the surge in popularity of diets such as the paleo diet, all meat contains excess complex protein and toxic hormones, chemicals and parasites. Many of the health benefits that those following the paleo diet seem to enjoy, notably weight loss, are as a result of what is absent in the diet – that is, processed grains and high fructose foods.

Eliminate fried food: Major chemical changes take place in food at the high temperatures generated by frying. Carcinogenic compounds can be created in the heated oil. Udo Erasmus, author of *Fats that Heal, Fats that Kill*, states that, if frying at all, we should only fry in water and add the oil afterwards once the food has cooled. For those transitioning off a lot of fried food, who still want that fatty feel that frying gives, the safest oil to fry in is coconut oil. The healthiest raw oils are the unhealthiest when they are heated to frying temperatures (for example olive oil). Follow the Mediterraneans and use olive oil on your salads, not in the frying pan.

Avoid the microwave: It is a massive generator of free radicals and causes considerable cellular degradation.

Avoid added salt: use celery instead.

Avoid alcohol, vinegar and soft drinks: they are unhealthy.

Avoid stress: Aim to eat only at times when you are calm and relaxed.

Fasting

I recommend adding a fasting day, one day a week, and every week. There are many benefits of fasting; I outline these in my e-book *Successful Fasting for Health and Vitality*, which provides a clear and easy-to-follow guide for getting the most from both short and longer fasts. This book is available via my website. Many people can't contemplate the idea of depriving themselves of food for even a day, let alone longer, but fasting is an excellent tool for health, so it would be a shame to miss out on some of these benefits. One fasting day a week rests the digestive system and causes no problems, although insulin-dependent diabetics, children, those more than 10 pounds underweight and pregnant women should seek medical advice first before embarking upon this practice, and would be best advised to avoid it altogether.

Increasing numbers of people are now being attracted to the concept of intermittent fasting, and this practice can have many benefits. In *The Fast Diet*, Dr Michael Mosley and Mimi Spencer relate that weight loss is only one benefit; the major ones are the reduced risk of degenerative diseases including diabetes, heart disease and cancer. The suspected, although not entirely proven, mode of action for this is via activation of Sirt-1, a gene which is part of the family of genes known as 'sirtuins'.

These 'longevity genes', when activated, switch our cells to survival, cell preservation and stress resistance mode, and while we all have them, whether they are active or not, can be greatly affected by our lifestyles. We can either activate them (thereby staying disease-free, and living a long, happy, active life), or switch them off (which leads to degeneration, pain and suffering). Here are a few things that will help to wake them up.

Caloric restriction

By caloric restriction, I don't mean starving yourself, but restricting calories while taking in optimal nutrition. There's a huge difference. This could mean conducting periodic fasts, or considering intermittent fasting (such as one or two days per week) as outlined in my book on fasting (see above).

Resveratrol

Resveratrol is a polyphenol compound found in dark-skinned fruit, for example grape skins, blueberries and blackberries. Just like other phytonutrients though, I would never recommend that anyone goes out and buys the latest resveratrol supplement, although as you can probably imagine, such things do exist. We are designed to eat food, not just a single one of the 25,000 antioxidants that are found in plants. By all means use a whole-food supplement that contains the foods high in resveratrol – this is what I do – but don't take resveratrol in isolation, since it may be oestrogenic (which would increase the risk of hormonally linked cancers such as breast, prostate and endometrial), and can also increase one's risk of bleeding. Additionally, a paper published in 2010 (Pacholec M, Bleasdale JE et al, 'SRT1720, SRT2183, SRT1460, and resveratrol are not direct activators of SIRT1', *Journal of Biological Chemistry*, 2010; 285(11): 8340-8351) indicated that resveratrol did not activate one particular type of sirtuin, so the benefits might not be 'across the board' anyway.

You should also be aware that resveratrol is not the only compound that has been found to activate our longevity genes, although it is the one we tend to hear most about at the moment. Quercetin (present in garlic and other bulbs), butein and fisetin share the same honour, as do unpronounceables such as piceatannol and isoliquiritigenin. Don't worry about the names. You can find all of these compounds in the food that you eat, but only if your diet is based on whole, unprocessed plants.

Once again, the research seems to be pointing to the same inescapable conclusions: a whole-food, plant-based diet is the best for us in every way.

Toxic exposure

This is a huge subject and beyond the scope of a general chapter such as this, but in chapter 5 the huge problem of environmental pollution was discussed. Why not spend a day having a look around your house, and maybe your work environment too? Think about all the things you come into contact with. What is in your bathroom cupboard? What are your clothes made of? What is in your personal care products? Consider replacing them with non-toxic ingredients. Have a look at your cleaning products. Is there anything there that has an 'irritant' symbol on it? It's time to change to a more natural and biodegradable type. How about the kitchen cupboards? Is there anything lurking in there that you know isn't good for you?

What is on your bed? Since we should ideally spend eight hours a day there, on average, what is it that is coming into contact with your skin? Make sure your sheets are organic cotton, not synthetic fibres; likewise with any night clothes that you wear.

Clear the clutter

In chapter 5 I wrote about clearing the mind with meditation. If your personal environment is cluttered and full of 'stuff', it can be a reflection of what is going on inside. Why not take a weekend to look at each room in your house? Is there anything there which you don't need or use?

According to Dr Roberta Lee, author of *The Superstress Solution*, research shows that we secrete more cortisol when we're surrounded by disarray, which, as outlined in chapters 5 and 9, is very bad news for the body. By having a good tidy-up, you can reclaim not only your surroundings but also your sense of calm. If it all seems a bit overwhelming, break it down into stages. Tackle one room at a time, or even, if things have got way out of hand, just a wardrobe. Sort out what you're going to keep and what is for recycling. Having a good clear-out is incredibly therapeutic and will have you feeling better about yourself in no time at all. Even just spending 20 minutes per week on housework can be enough to reduce depression by 20 per cent, according to a 2009 study (Hamer M, Stamatakis E, Steptoe A, 'Dose-response relationship between physical activity and mental health: the Scottish Health Survey', *British Journal of Sports Medicine* 2009; 43: 1111-1114).

Rest

For most people seven to eight hours of rest is usually needed, and it is very important not to get into a situation of 'sleep debt'. Studies reported in *Scientific American* show that such short-term sleep deprivation leads to a foggy brain, worsened vision, impaired driving, and trouble remembering. Long-term effects include obesity, insulin resistance and heart disease. Many people suffer from chronic sleep deprivation. Both the number of hours you sleep and the intensity of that sleep are important.

Deprive someone of REM sleep for more than a few consecutive nights and psychosis can rapidly ensue. Sleep debt can be repaid, but it takes time. The greatest benefits seem to be obtained by regularly getting to bed half an hour to an hour earlier, rather than getting up three hours later than normal at the weekend. Remember the improved mental and physical capabilities that come with being well rested, and maybe that late-night movie, or extra hours of work, will seem less attractive.

Positive environment and thinking

Positive thinking could be the greatest health-creator that we have at our disposal. Indeed, *The Power of Positive Thinking* by Norman Vincent Peale, published as long ago as 1952, suggests that we can overcome anything we put our minds to, and it has now been scientifically proven that optimistic people live longer than pessimists. A study published in the January 2012 issue of the journal *Psychosomatic Medicine* showed that optimism was a significant predictor of longevity. Research points to the relationship between optimism and rates of depression, lower levels of distress, greater resistance to the common cold and reduced risk of death from cardiovascular disease. Optimism will therefore be positively affecting your immune system, nervous system and circulatory system for starters. And think of the knock-on effects of that.

Be positive, taking responsibility for your life's circumstances. See every opportunity as a chance to progress and grow. Create health by envisioning it. Focus on that vision before you go to bed. Learn to love who you are. Why not create a self-esteem journal, and every evening before you go to bed, write down seven things that you like about yourself? Every three months, read over what you have written and see how much better it makes you feel.

Surround yourself with positive, happy people and avoid the energy-drainers. This might be easier said than done to start with, but you attract what you put out to the universe. Start being more happy and optimistic and more of that is likely to come your way. You are reading this book for a reason, and my guess is that you're already positive and happy. Let's create more of the same, and light up the world with a message of joy and hope.

What lies behind us and what lies before us are tiny matters compared to what lies within us.

It's within you! Stay well.

Summary

- Incorporate some sprouted food into your diet
- Enjoy a green juice every day
- Eat organic food
- Avoid fried food
- Add a fasting day to your routine
- Reduce your exposure to toxicity wherever possible
- Clear the clutter
- Ensure that you get adequate rest
- Develop and cultivate positivity in your life.

Appendix 1

Is supplementation necessary?

Food supplements have been around for many years, and now there are literally thousands of types and many different brands on the market. What do we need, if indeed we need anything at all? I think the supplements debate is one that will be ongoing for many years to come. How do we know who to believe, when we hear one expert saying that they are essential and another who vehemently believes that we can get everything from a so-called 'balanced diet', whatever their personal interpretation of that happens to be?

When I approach any matter that is open to debate, I like to take a logical and scientific perspective rather than an emotional one. So, firstly, do we actually need to supplement? Practitioners from the Natural Hygiene movement (those who base their diet upon tropical fruit and green leaves) state that we should never do so, and that all supplements are toxic at a cellular level and that no animal in the wild needs to supplement, so why should humans differ? I would love to agree, but that would imply that we are living in a perfect world, which we are not. In my opinion, we would have to be living somewhere with no air pollution, no water pollution, no environmental pollution, no cities, no commercial agriculture and no soil depletion. We would have to be living in small groups in a tropical forest, eating pure food from nature's bounty. Heaven! Sadly, with possibly very few exceptions, I think those days are over.

At the time of writing, 80 per cent of the global population lives in cities, with their fast pace of life, overcrowding, pollution and other stressors to well-being. Food is shipped to such cities from all parts of the world, and is often grown in mineral-depleted soil. Here in the UK, if we rely on home-produced agriculture, we have to be aware that the soil is almost totally devoid of selenium, and this is only one of the 90 or so minerals that we need for optimal health. If food is being brought in from afar, it has to be picked before it is fully ripe to avoid spoilage, which further compromises its nutritional status. The change from a more plant-based to a meat-based diet over the past 100 years (USDA Economic Research Service, 2008) has led to further challenges to our micronutrition, and fewer antioxidants and phytonutrients being consumed.

You can probably guess from the above that I am an advocate of food supplementation. You'd be right. There is still one element of the world's population, however, that in my opinion, would not require any supplements. These very healthy and fortunate people would be living the following lifestyle:

- They would live between 30 degrees north and 30 degrees south of the equator
- They would expose their skin to the sun for 30 minutes every day
- They would exercise for 30 to 60 minutes per day
- They would have absolutely no negative stress in their lives, since stress, as we have learned, increases the demand for certain minerals and antioxidants
- They would be eating a diet based on fresh vegetables, leafy greens and ripe tropical fruit, and would addition-ally be making green juice every day, which would contain the sprouted foods such as sunflower greens and pea shoots. They would also utilise wheatgrass juice
- They would grow their own food in mineral-rich soil that is watered with rain and spring water. That soil would

contain all the minerals that are known to be essential for exceptional health.

This in itself is a pretty tall order, but there's more:

- They would also be meditating for 20 minutes per day to tune in with nature and their life's purpose
- They would breathe pure, unpolluted air and drink spring water from a spring, not a plastic bottle.

Once they had been doing this for two years, there would be no further need, in my opinion, for supplements.

If this sums up your lifestyle, I would genuinely love to meet you!

History

Let's take a brief look now at the history of the supplements industry. The original food supplements were medicinal herbs. These would have been locally sourced from woods and fields close to home. They would be fresh, or dried and taken as teas, and would bring about a positive change in those taking them. They had a very high safety margin. In effect, they were potentiated foods, or food-medicine. They were bitter, and therefore people couldn't eat a lot of them. This prevented over-consumption, which potentially could have led to adverse effects.

Dried herbs and bitter greens were then encapsulated and given as supplements. This was successful, so led on to the mass expansion of the synthetic supplement boom, largely driven by the pharmaceutical industry. Check the labels of many synthetic supplements and you will find that they are made by one of the pharmaceutical companies. Over 95 per cent of the supplements on the market today are synthetic, and this goes for the ones in the 'good' health stores too. Synthetic supplements are of no value whatsoever from a health perspective. This is a strong statement, so allow me to elaborate.

I'd like to give just one example of a synthetic supplement compared with a food-derived supplement and what we can expect to see regarding the benefits of each, and if either could be potentially harmful. I'll choose something that we are all familiar with – vitamin C. I haven't chosen this because I feel it is the most important nutrient – far from it. I have chosen it because it was one of the first to be discovered, and there is more published research on vitamin C than all other nutrients. Vitamin C is essential to human health, and it first came to light when the vitamin C in citrus fruit was found to prevent scurvy in 19th-century sailors. Unlike most mammals, humans have lost the metabolic pathway by which biosynthesis of vitamin C can take place. We share this enzyme deficiency with the guinea pig and the fruit bat, so all three of our species require a dietary source.

Mention vitamin C and most people think of oranges. That is good, because at least they are not thinking of pills. Vitamin C is best described as vitamin C complex, since it is composed of eight potent antioxidants enclosed by an outer shell, which protects the central elements. I like to give the analogy of a Malteser to describe this. For those who have never had one, Maltesers are spherical sweets with an inner honeycomb centre and an outer chocolate shell. The outer chocolate shell of the Malteser is like the ascorbic acid part of vitamin C complex, and acts as the antioxidant for the important central parts, and the honeycomb centre represents the remaining eight factors. Ascorbic acid is *not* the same as vitamin C, just as a chocolate shell is *not* a Malteser. (This is only an analogy – please be aware that Maltesers are not a source of vitamin C.) This is a very important point, since many people think that ascorbic acid is the same as vitamin C, whereas it is in no way the same as the complex that you would get from oranges, or camu camu berries, for that matter.

Supplements containing ascorbic acid should be avoided. Not only is it not vitamin C, it is cheaply made by boiling up coal tar and sulphuric acid. It is only one ninth of real vitamin C complex. How can it possibly be the same as that found in fruit and berries? Not only has it no benefits, it is harmful, especially if taken in mega-doses for long periods (such as, 1000 to 2000 mg daily), which is what some practitioners still suggest. Taken in this way, synthetic ascorbic acid acidifies, drives minerals out of the bones and damages the kidneys, all the while not giving any of the benefits associated with food-source vitamin C complex. The reason it seems to make people 'feel better' is as a result of its stimulant effect upon the adrenal glands, which is not the same as creating health. We could derive the same 'benefit' from a strong cup of coffee, with the same detrimental effects. It is like taking a whip to a tired horse. Don't do it.

This is just one example of what happens when we try to outsmart nature. I believe it was Thomas Edison who said, 'Until man can replicate a blade of grass, we can laugh at his so-called scientific achievements.' How can anyone think that they can boil up coal tar and sulphuric acid and create oranges? Not a chance.

In 1998, there were approximately 12,000 phytonutrients that had been discovered by science. Some interesting ones are lutein, zeaxanthin and resveratrol, but we now know that there are over 25,000 of these beneficial substances in plants. Look on the ingredients listing of a synthetic supplement and you will see a list of maybe 20 ingredients if you're lucky. Where are you going to get the remaining 24,980? And what about all those that we don't even know about yet? We need these beneficial nutrients, for sure, but it's important to state that we need them in the same ratios that they are found in nature, not those that are guessed at in a lab.

Some supplements are starting to hit the shelves that state on the label that they are 'food-source', but I believe that these should be avoided too if there are only a few ingredients listed. Remember, we need thousands.

My next statement is therefore that any supplement we take has to be made from whole plants. Here are some questions that we should be asking of supplement manufacturers:

1. How has the supplement been produced? This is of vital importance. If it has been synthetically prepared from individual, isolated ingredients, rather than being extracted from whole plants, it will be of very limited value.

2. How has the supplement been processed? If it is made from whole plants, but has been processed at high temperatures, the heat-labile factors such as the phyto-nutrients we have just been discussing will have been denatured and therefore will be of no value.

3. Is the supplement bioavailable? In other words, when you take it, has it been demonstrated to get into the blood stream, or to the organs by which it is needed? If bioavailability studies have been performed, where are they published? Have they, for example, been published in a peer-reviewed scientific journal?

4. Has the research been performed on this particular supplement, or has it, for example, been performed on an ingredient which is present in the supplement, and therefore only assumed that this supplement will have the same effect?

5. Has the supplement itself been tested on humans, or a different species? We cannot always extrapolate studies in rats to give us information on benefits for humans.

6. Are there any adverse side effects known from the use of this supplement? If so, where are the results published?

If you can't get answers to these questions, there probably are no studies. Supplement manufacturers should be doing this sort of research as a matter of course in my opinion. Remember, plants can take up minerals from the soil and incorporate them into their structure. Humans cannot.

Once you have found what looks like a good whole-food supplement, it is time to drill a little deeper. The human diet, as I have discussed in this book, should be based on the green foods since they are the most mineral-rich. However, great as they are, greens do not contain all of the phytonutrients that are present in plants of other colours. No one plant has them all. For example, resveratrol, highly prized in current research for its benefits for cardiovascular health, its anticancer properties and its potential for the enhancement of longevity, is only present in foods that are dark red and purple/blue, such as dark grapes and blueberries. Ideally our whole-food supplement should contain plants of the whole spectrum of colours. With regard to the processing of that supplement, juicing the raw ingredients will most likely lead to better bioavailability of the phytonutrients, since any fibre content could hinder absorption. In other parts of this book, I have recommended certain specific supplements because they fulfil these important criteria.

In summary, almost everyone can benefit from supplementation, provided it is based on whole-foods: if you're already healthy, you'll get healthier. If you're ill, you'll help yourself at a cellular level to improve. After all, there is no known disease process that is not aided by better nutrition.

Appendix 2

Juice Plus studies

The following summarises the research findings that support the benefits of the Juice PLUS+ supplementation that I have used for 19 years, and which I recommend to my clients.

Juice PLUS+® delivers key phytonutrients that are absorbed by the body

Investigators at the University of South Carolina,[1] Tokyo Women's Medical University[2] and the Medical University of Vienna[3] studied the bioavailability (absorption by the body) of select nutrients found in Juice PLUS+® and concluded that Juice PLUS+® effectively increases antioxidant nutrients and folate. Other published studies have also shown various phytonutrients in Juice PLUS+® are bioavailable. These studies were conducted by independent researchers from the Georgetown/UCLA,[4] University of Sydney in Australia,[5] King's College in London,[6] Brigham Young University,[7] the University of Arizona,[8] the University of Florida[9] and the University of Texas Health Science Center[10].

Juice PLUS+® reduces oxidative stress

Several of these studies which included various aspects of nutrient bioavailability[1, 2, 6, 9, 10] also reported improved antioxidant enzyme levels, plasma antioxidant capacity and reduced lipid peroxides, a key indicator of oxidative stress. In addition, researchers at the Medical University of Graz, Austria[11, 12] and the University of North Carolina, Greensboro[13, 14] found that Juice PLUS+® Fruit, Vegetable and Vineyard Blends together were effective in reducing a marker for oxidative stress associated with aerobic exercise.

Juice PLUS+® can help with systemic inflammation

Chronic inflammation is common. Emerging science is identifying different markers of generalised inflammation, even in otherwise healthy people. Published clinical research from the University of South Carolina[1] demonstrated Juice PLUS+® reduces several of these markers.

Juice PLUS+® can help maintain a healthy immune system and DNA integrity

Good nutrition is important for the normal function of the immune system and healthy DNA. Published clinical research indicated that Juice PLUS+® supports several measures of immune function – in law school students at the University of Florida[9] and in elderly people in a study conducted at the University of Arizona.[8] A study of healthcare professionals at Charité University Medical Centre in Berlin,[15] Germany, reported Juice PLUS+® use over the cold winter months resulted in a 20 per cent reduction in moderate/severe symptom days.

Studies conducted have shown a reduction in DNA damage after taking Juice PLUS+® in the law students at the University of Florida[9] and in an elderly population at Brigham Young University.[7]

Juice PLUS+® positively affects several key indicators of cardiovascular wellness

Studies have been carried out into the effect of Juice PLUS+® on several markers of heart and vascular health:

- **Homocysteine** is an amino acid that is found in the blood. Maintaining healthy homocysteine levels is thought to be important for the heart and cardiovascular system. A clinical study at the University of Sydney in Australia[5] reported a reduction in homocysteine levels – even though the levels of the Australian subjects were already within an acceptable range. Researchers in Foggia, Italy[16] also found a reduction in homocysteine levels in people with elevated levels of homocysteine.
- Researchers at the University of Maryland School of Medicine[17] found that subjects who consumed Juice PLUS+® were better able to maintain the normal **elasticity of arteries**, even after a high-fat meal.
- Investigators at Vanderbilt University School of Medicine18 monitored **several measures of vascular health** in a low-risk population who took Juice PLUS+® for two years and noted various improvements with no adverse side effects.

Additional published results

Two pilot studies – one on the role of Juice PLUS+® in pregnancy health[19] and one on the effect of Juice PLUS+® on oxidative stress in smokers[20] – are now being followed up with placebo-controlled double-blind clinical trials.

References

1. Jin Y, et al, 'Systemic inflammatory load in humans is suppressed by consumption of two formulations of dried, encapsulated juice concentrate', *Molecular Nutrition & Food Research* 2010; 54: 1-9.

2. Kawashima A, et al, 'Four week supplementation with mixed fruit and vegetable juice concentrates increased protective serum antioxidants and folate and decreased plasma homocysteine in Japanese subjects', *Asia Pacific Journal of Clinical Nutrition* 2007; 16(3): 411-421.

3. Kiefer I, et al, 'Supplementation with mixed fruit and vegetable juice concentrates increased serum antioxidants and folate in healthy adults', *Journal of the American College of Nutrition* 2004; 23(3): 205-211.

4. Wise JA, et al, 'beta-carotene and alpha-tocopherol in healthy overweight adults; depletion kinetics are correlated with adiposity', *International Journal of Food Science and Nutrition* 2009; 60(S3): 65-75

5. Samman S, et al, 'A mixed fruit and vegetable concentrate increases plasma antioxidant vitamins and folate and lowers plasma homocysteine in men', *Journal of Nutrition* 2003; 133(7): 2188-2193.

6. Leeds AR, et al, 'Availability of micronutrients from dried, encapsulated fruit and vegetable preparations: a study in healthy volunteers', *Journal of Human Nutrition and Dietetics* 2000; 13(1): 21-27.

7. Smith MJ, et al, 'Supplementation with fruit and vegetable extracts may decrease DNA damage in the peripheral lymphocytes of an elderly population', *Nutrition Research* 1999; 19(10): 1507-1518.

8. Inserra PF, et al, 'Immune function in elderly smokers and nonsmokers improves during supplementation with fruit and vegetable extracts', *Integrative Medicine* 1999;2(1): 3-10.

9. Nantz MP, et al, 'Immunity and antioxidant capacity in humans is enhanced by consumption of a dried, encapsulated fruit and vegetable juice concentrate', *Journal of Nutrition* 2006; 136(10): 2606-2610.

10. Wise JA, et al, 'Changes in plasma carotenoid, alpha-tocopherol, and lipid peroxide levels in response to

supplementation with concentrated fruit and vegetable extracts: a pilot study', *Current Therapeutic Research* 1996; 57(6): 445-4619.

11. Lamprecht M, et al, 'Several indicators of oxidative stress, immunity, and illness improved in trained men consuming an encapsulated juice powder concentrate for 28 weeks', *Journal of Nutrition* 2007; 137(12): 2737-2741.

12. Lamprecht M, et al, 'Protein modification responds to exercise intensity and antioxidant supplementation', *Medicine & Science in Sports & Exercise* 2009; 41(1): 155-163.

13. Bloomer RJ, et al, 'Oxidative stress response to aerobic exercise: comparison of antioxidant supplements', *Medicine & Science in Sports & Exercise* 2006; 38 (6): 1098-1105.

14. Goldfarb AH, et al, 'Effects of a Fruit/Berry/Vegetable supplement on muscle function and oxidative stress', *Medicine and Science in Sports and Exercise* 2011; 43(3): 501-508. DOI: 10.1249/MSS.0b013e3181f1ef48.

15. Roll S, et al, 'Reduction of common cold symptoms by encapsulated juice powder concentrate of fruits and vegetables: a randomized, double-blind, placebo-controlled trial', *British Journal of Nutrition* 2011; 105: 118-122.

16. Panunzio MF, et al, 'Supplementation with fruit and vegetable concentrate decreases plasma homocysteine levels in a dietary controlled trial', *Nutrition Research* 2003; 23(9): 1221-1228.

17. Plotnick GD, et al, 'Effect of supplemental phytonutrients on impairment of the flow-mediated brachial artery vasoactivity after a single high-fat meal', *Journal of the American College of Cardiology* 2003; 41(10): 1744-1749.

18. Houston MC, et al, 'Juice powder concentrate and systemic blood pressure, progression of coronary artery calcium and antioxidant status in hypertensive subjects: a pilot study', *eCAM* 2007; 4(4): 455-462.

19. Odom CD, et al, 'Phytonutrients may decrease obstetric

complications; a retrospective study', *Journal of the American Nutraceutical Association* 2006; 9(1): 23-27.

20. Bamonti F, et al, 'Increased free malondialdehyde concentrations in smokers normalise with a mixed fruit and vegetable juice concentrate; a pilot study', *Clinical Chemistry and Laboratory Medicine* 2006; 44(4): 391-395.

Hospitals and universities that investigated or are investigating Juice PLUS+®

Brigham Young University, USA
Charité University, Berlin, Germany
Georgetown University, USA
King's College, London, England
Medical University of Graz, Austria
Medical University of Vienna, Austria
Tokyo Women's Medical University, Japan
University of Arizona, USA
University of Birmingham, England
University of California, Los Angeles, USA
University of Florida, USA
University of Maryland School of Medicine, USA
University of Milan, Italy
University of Mississippi Medical Center, USA
University of North Carolina-Greensboro, USA
University of South Carolina, USA
University of Sydney, Australia
University of Texas Health Science Center, USA
University of Texas/MD Anderson, USA
University of Würzburg, Germany
Vanderbilt University School of Medicine, USA
Wake Forest University, USA (with the NCI-National Institutes of Health)
Yale University-Griffin Hospital Prevention Research Center, USA

Appendix 3

Resources

My website
For personal consultations, group classes, seminars, books, e-books, CD & MP3 recordings, and free monthly newsletter
www.therawfoodscientist.com

UK-based living/raw food retreat
I run and teach at this popular retreat twice a year in Gloucestershire, UK. Why not come and join me?
www.rawfoodretreat.eu

Fasting retreat in the UK
Health Etcetera, Winchester
www.healthetcetera.com

Aconbury Sprouts
For home delivery of sprouted food and seeds in the UK
www.wheatgrass-uk.com

Got Sprouts
In the USA, try Got Sprouts for sprouted food and seeds
www.GotSprouts.com

The Fresh Network
For everything relating to the living foods lifestyle: books, DVDs,

CDs, juicers, dehydrators, sprouting equipment and raw foods both in the UK and internationally, see the banner link on my website shop page

www.therawfoodscientist.com/Shop.htm

Sunfood

For similar foods to the Fresh Network in the USA and Canada
www.sunfood.com

Discount Juicers

For juicers, blenders and dehydrators and other kitchen equipment in the USA
www.discountjuicers.com

Upaya Naturals

For juicers, blenders and living foods in Canada
www.upayanaturals.com
416-617-3096

Antidote for Modern Living

UK suppliers of the Hippocrates Health Institute range of food supplements, including vitamin B12 (see chapter 5) and vitamin D3 (chapters 6, 9, 10 and 11) and the HHIZyme supplemental enzymes as mentioned in chapter 2.
www.antidoteformodernliving.co.uk

Kiki Health

Under the same ownership as The Fresh Network, Kiki Health sells enzymes, probiotics and other supplements, including E3Live liquid blue-green algae, as mentioned in chapter 2, page 60. They also stock natural toxin-free hair and body care products. Highly recommended.
www.kiki-health.com

Infinity Foods
UK wholesalers stocking many of the goods that are supplied to health stores. I buy all my nuts, seeds, seaweeds, nut butters, prepared raw crackers and many other raw foods from Infinity. They also sell body care products, laundry and cleaning products in bulk. Minimum order value applies.
www.infinityfoods.co.uk

Raw Power (Australia)
For juicers, blenders, dehydrators, books, superfoods and all things related to living foods lifestyle, in Australia
www.rawpower.com.au

Australian Wheatgrass (Australia)
For home delivery of wheatgrass for juicing, and for seeds and sprouters, in the Sydney area
www.wheatgrass.com.au

The Wheatgrass Company (Australia)
For similar, in the Melbourne area
www.wheatgrass.com.au

Living Foods Lifestyle (New Zealand)
For kitchen and sprouting equipment, and books
www.livingfoodslifestyle.co.nz

Juicers (New Zealand)
For juicers and blenders
www.juicersnewzealand.co.nz

Keith's Wheatgrass (New Zealand)
For home delivery of wheatgrass in the Auckland area
www.keithswheatgrass.co.nz

Meditation CD
By Chrissy White
http://chrissywhitecom.moonfruit.com/#/store/4567333498

Juice Plus
The supplement I recommend: available worldwide via the following site
http://mt016459.juiceplus.com

Recommended health establishments

Hippocrates Health Institute
Based in Florida, their three-week Life Transformation Program is, in my opinion, the best there is. If you're considering a visit, contact me via max@therawfoodscientist.com to receive a gift card to use during your stay.
www.hippocratesinst.org

Tree of Life
Based in Arizona, the Tree of Life offers spiritual approach to living food
www.treeoflife.nu

Recommended reading

The China Study, by T Colin Campbell. (Published by Ben Bella, 2006)

Living Foods for Optimum Health: staying healthy in an unhealthy world, by Brian Clement. (Published by Prima Life, 1998)

Food IS Medicine: The Scientific Evidence, by Brian Clement. (Published by the Book Publishing Company. Vol 1: 2012, Vol 2: 2013)

Sprouts: The Miracle Food, by Steve Meyerowitz. (Published by the Book Publishing Company, 1999)

Life Force: Superior Health and Longevity, by Brian Clement. (Published by Healthy Living Publications, 2007)

Killer Fish: how eating aquatic life endangers your health, by Brian Clement. (Published by the Book Publishing Company, 2012)

There is a Cure for Diabetes, by Gabriel Cousens. (Published by North Atlantic Books, 2013)

Healthy at 100, by John Robbins. (Published by Ballantine Books Inc, 2007)

Diet for a New America (25th anniversary edition), by John Robbins. (Published by HJ Kramer/New World Library, 2012)

Eating for Beauty, by David Wolfe. (Published by North Atlantic Books, 2008)

Deep Feeling, Deep Healing: The Heart, Mind and Soul of Getting Well, by Andy Bernay-Roman. (Published by Spectrum Healing Press, 2002 – out of print)

Top 10 Raw Food Tips for Osteoporosis, by Max Tuck. (Available from Amazon Media and www.therawfoodscientist.com, 2011)

Raw Food Made Simple, by Karen Knowler. (Published by Raw Food Coach Media, 2010)

Recommended recipe books

The Raw Gourmet by Nomi Shannon. (Published by Alive Books, 2007)

Healthful Cuisine – accessing the lifeforce within you through raw and living foods by Anna-Maria Clement and Kelly Serbonich. (Published by Book Publishing, 2008)

Rainbow Green Live Food Cuisine by Dr Gabriel Cousens. (Published by North Atlantic Books, 2003)

Good Raw Food Recipes – delicious raw and living food for energy and wellness by Judy Barber. (Published by Rethink Press, 2012)

Recommended equipment

You can get by with minimal equipment when you first switch to a more plant-based diet, but after a while you will need to invest in some kitchen equipment to enable you to get the greatest benefits from this way of eating. The equipment you buy will depend on your budget, so I have subdivided this section into those pieces that really are almost essential, some that are very useful, and others that are just 'nice to have'. All of this equipment can be found via the companies listed above.

(Almost) essential

A good juicer. I recommend the Green Star Elite, but it is expensive (£550). A more economical juicer would be the single-gear Omega 8006 juicer, which is approximately half the price of the Green Star. I absolutely do not recommend a cheap centrifugal juicer. It won't do wheatgrass, it won't do greens, it is hard to clean and you will rapidly get fed up with it. Save your money until you can afford one of the above models. For a really cheap wheatgrass juicer, try the Z-star, a hand-turning juicer that will juice other things as well, just to get you started. Remember, a good juicer doesn't just juice things. You can make a whole array of food in it, since the good models come with a 'blank screen' attachment which allows you to homogenise food. With this attachment, you can make anything from pâtés to baby food to ice cream.

Sprouting jars. These are essential to get you started with growing your own sprouts. They are cheap and can be used over and over again. For travelling, try a sprouting bag; it's light and won't break in your luggage.

Blender. You can get by with a cheap blender or liquidiser – I did for years, but it is good to have a high-powered blender so that you can make soups, nut milks and dressings. The best (and most expensive) blender is the Vitamix Vita-Prep 3 (£697), but once you own one, you will wonder how you ever managed without it. Cheaper than the Vitamix range of blenders, but almost as good, is the JTC OmniBlend range (from £229). Blenders can be bought for as little as £40 and they will usually be quite adequate initially. It's also a good idea to check out second-hand machines.

Seed trays. These are useful if you are going to grow your own wheatgrass and tray greens at home, but not essential – you can have your sprouts home delivered from, for example, Aconbury in the UK, or Got Sprouts in the USA.

Water filtration system. See chapter 8 for why we need good quality water to drink.

Some good chef's knives. I recommend ceramic knives of differing sizes – three should suffice. Mine are made by Viners and Kyocera. Try an internet search for a supplier in your country.

Very useful

A dehydrator. I managed for years before buying one of these machines second hand. The best type of dehydrator is the Excalibur. Mine is a 9-tray version; you can also get a smaller 5-tray design. It is used for making crackers and drying previously soaked nuts and seeds. It can also be used for warming food. It's great for anyone who likes their food with a crispy texture. Excalibur dehydrators cost from £149 for a 5-tray model.

Automatic sprouter. I now wouldn't be without this piece of kit, but I managed for years with just growing my sprouts in jars. I use the Easy Green machine (approx £189), but started off with the Fresh Life sprouter (£129). The Fresh Life is good because it doesn't take up much space, but the motor on mine gave up after two years of regular use. The Easy Green is a more robust machine but it does take up more space on the kitchen worktop.

Food processor. I have a Magimix food processor (approx £200), which is incredibly useful. I use it for chopping nuts, grating vegetables and you can also make soup in it if you don't have a blender.

Nice to have

Vegetable spiraliser. This fun machine will turn vegetables into different-sized spirals, and it is generally used to make 'spaghetti' out of courgettes or other vegetables. If you have children who won't eat their vegetables, using a spiraliser, and getting them to help you, might just spark their interest. It is also a great machine to use for making attractive garnishes when holding dinner parties.

Unusual ingredients

Some of the foods or ingredients suggested in this book may be unfamiliar to you, so I have given a list below outlining the benefits of their use. You can find most of these foods online, from sites such as the Fresh Network (see above) in the UK, Sunfood in the USA and Canada, or at a good independent local health store.

Almond butter/other nut butters: These are made by grinding unroasted almonds or other nuts into a paste. A large amount of heat can be generated in the grinding process, so it is best to use a brand that ensures they grind the nuts in small batches to minimise heating. In the UK, I use Carley's nut and seed butters, which are available from the Fresh Network and Infinity Foods.

Braggs Liquid Aminos: A salty condiment used in sauces and dressings. It is sold in most good health stores. Raw tamari, or Nama Shoyu, are substitutes for Braggs.

Carob powder: A powder that comes from raw carob pods, carob powder is a good substitute for chocolate powder in any raw recipe. Most carob powder is roasted. Make sure you get the raw version.

Chia seeds: These tiny black seeds are a true superfood. High in essential fats and protein, you will need chia seeds for the recipe at the end of chapter 3, page 49.

Hemp seeds: High in protein and essential fats, hemp seeds can be used in salads. Sprinkle them into soups and smoothies too.

Maca: A ground Andean root, raw maca is adaptogenic and is great for people suffering from stress. Find it via the Fresh Network and Sunfood (see above).

Miso: Miso is a fermented soya product and is used in some recipes to give a salty taste and a smooth texture. Find it in health stores. It lasts one month after opening if kept in a sealed container and refrigerated.

Seaweed: Seaweeds are fantastically rich in minerals. Try flat raw nori sheets to make wraps and raw vegan sushi rolls. Other types of seaweed include dulse, hijiki, wakame and khombu. Rinse the dry seaweed before use (except nori) to remove excess salt. I use the Clearspring brand, available in good health stores, via Infinity Foods and the Fresh Network.

Stevia: A zero-calorie powdered sweetener that causes no blood sugar irregularities and comes from a plant leaf, rather than being chemically manufactured, stevia is now available in the UK in good health stores and also via the Fresh Network. Use very little in your recipes and drinks – it's incredibly sweet.

Sunwarrior protein powder: A top-quality raw vegan protein product that I recommend for athletes, people who have difficulty keeping weight on, and those wishing to gain muscle mass. Made from fermented brown rice, it is stocked by the Fresh Network in the UK, and Sunfood in the USA and Canada, to name but two suppliers. It is easy to find stockists online. Mix it into smoothies after exercising.

Tahini: Raw tahini is a great source of calcium. It is made from ground, unroasted sesame seeds. I use the Carley's brand, as per almond butter above. Use it in soups, smoothies and dressings.

Tamari: A salty, fermented soya sauce used in dressings and as a seasoning. I recommend using only small quantities due to the potential oestrogenic effects of soya as described in chapter 9, although fermented soya appears to be less problematic in this regard.

Index

Index

bioavailability of supplements, 180
bioflavonoids/flavonols, 35, 58, 107
birth control pills, 110
bisphenol-A, 104–105
bladder cancer and garlic, 107
blender, 193–194
blood, 52–57
    filtering, 62
    oxygen carriage in and delivery to
    tissues, 51, 52, 54, 56, 96
    red cells, 51, 53, 54, 62, 75
    white cells, 53, 62, 88, 92, 93, 107
blood vessels *see* arteries; vascular
    health
blue-green algae *see* algae
blueberries, 58, 147–148, 154, 164
bone, 134–136, 149
bowel *see* intestine
Braggs Liquid Aminos, 196
brain, 65
    factors adversely affecting, 69
    foods, 72–75
    oxygen and, 66
breakfast suggestions, 162–165
breast cancer
    root canal treatment and, 24
    soya and, 124
breathing
    abdominal/deep, 66, 97, 101, 163
    fresh air, 96, 97

cabbage, 38
cadmium, 78, 79
caffeine, 35, 58, 97, 106, 112, 141
calcium, foods high in, 73
caloric restriction, 170
cancer, 5–6
    alcohol and, 31–32
    bladder, garlic and, 107
    bowel, 11, 43
    breast *see* breast cancer
    hormones in food and, 130
    stomach, 22
    see also carcinogens
carbohydrates
    in food combining, 15, 17
    metabolism, MSM supplements
    and, 150
    sprouted, 161

    see also oligosaccharides; starch;
    sugar
carcinogens, 10, 31, 35, 37, 38, 43, 79,
    138, 146, 156, 168
cardiovascular system *see* circulatory
    system
carob powder, 196
carrot, 35
cayenne pepper, 59
    lemon water and, 21, 55, 162
celery in juices, 19
central nervous system, 55, 72, 116,
    128
cereal(s) and grains, 72
    by-products, 44
    sprouted, 161
    whole grain, 37
cereal grasses, 52
chewing, 14
chia seed, 164–165, 196
    porridge, 49–50, 165
chlorine in drinking water, 104
chlorophyll, 20, 21, 35, 52, 53, 56, 66,
    74
chocolate, 57–58
    Carob powder as substitute, 196
cholesterol, 4, 7, 29–30, 33, 115, 118,
    120
    bad, 33, 35
    lowering, 11, 33, 35, 44, 47, 59, 92
chondroitin sulphate, 155–156
circulatory (cardiovascular) system,
    53–64
    factors affecting, 55
    foods for, 57–60
    Juice Plus and, 184
    recipe for, 63
citric acid (Krebs) cycle, 27–28
citrus fruits, 37–38, 58, 178
coconut and cranberry juice, 108
coconut oil, 118, 168
cod liver oil, 155
coffee, 67, 106, 108, 179
cold water immersion, immune
    stimulation by, 91–92
colon
    healthy, requirements for, 47–48
    hydrotherapy/enema, 32–33, 34,
    48–49

Index

fenugreek sprouts, 161
fermented foods, 7, 18, 38, 87
  miso, 196
  soya, 124
  tamari, 197
fibre, dietary, 11, 43–44
  insoluble, 44, 47
  oestrogenic compounds and, 110, 112
  soluble, 44, 47
fish oil, 59, 60, 144, 152
  see also cod liver oil
flavourings in sports drinks, 137
flax oil, 7, 60
flax water, 33
fluoride, 25
food(s)
  basic recommendations, 167–169
  combining, 15–19
   good vs poor, 16
  green *see* green foods/vegetables
  for healthy brain, 72–75
  for healthy circulation, 57–60
  for healthy liver, 34–37
  for healthy skin, 147–150
  for healthy urinary system, 97, 106–108
  hormones in, 130, 130
  plant *see* plant foods
  raw *see* raw food
  sulphur-containing, 150
  supplements *see* supplements
  see also diet
food processor, 195
free radicals, 58, 82, 94, 117, 142–143, 152, 153, 169
  see also oxidative stress
Fresh Network, The, 188
fried food, 168
fructose, 116–117, 137
fruit, 9–10
  acid *see* acid fruit
  citrus, 37–38, 58, 178
  dried, 70, 116
  in food combining, 16

gall bladder, 29–30, 47
  flush (and liver), 30, 32–34, 39
GALT (gut-associated lymphatic

tissue), 87
garlic, 20, 34, 59, 90, 155
  circulation and, 59
  immune system and, 90
  liver/gallbladder flush and, 32, 34
  urinary system and, 107
gastric... *see* stomach
gastrointestinal system *see* digestive system
genetically-modified crops, 123
ginger, 21, 59, 154
gingko biloba, 59
gland, digestive tract, 13, 14
glucosamine, 155–156
glucose in sports drinks, 137
gluten, 43–44, 124–125
glycaemic index, low, 67, 164
glycation, 117, 152
Got Sprouts, 188
grains *see* cereals
grape(s), 56, 58, 108
grapefruit, 35, 147–148
green foods/vegetables, 66, 161–162
  dark, 148
  leafy, 8, 16, 35–36, 43, 66, 104
  green juices, 19–21, 56, 70, 140, 141, 147, 163–164, 176
green tea, 35, 106, 112
grey hair, 157, 159
grounding, 131
group drumming, 93
growth hormone in food, 130
gut *see* digestive system

haeme, 53
haemoglobin, 51, 52, 53, 163
hair, 149, 156–157
  grey, 157, 159
happiness, 69, 71, 88
Hashimoto's thyroiditis, 117
Hay diet, 15
head massage, 157
Health Etcetera fasting retreat, 188
healthy diet, constituents, 1–11
heart, 51
  disease, 2, 4–5
  healthy, foods for, 58, 59
heavy metals, 137
  detoxification, 79, 163, 166

Index